Family-Centred Assessment and Intervention in Pediatric Rehabilitation

Family-Centred Assessment and Intervention in Pediatric Rehabilitation has been co-published simultaneously as *Physical & Occupational Therapy in Pediatrics*, Volume 18, Number 1 1998.

Family-Centred Assessment and Intervention in Pediatric Rehabilitation

Mary Law
Editor

Family-Centred Assessment and Intervention in Pediatric Rehabilitation has been co-published simultaneously as *Physical & Occupational Therapy in Pediatrics*, Volume 18, Number 1 1998.

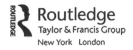

Routledge
Taylor & Francis Group
New York   London

Family-Centred Assessment and Intervention in Pediatric Rehabilitation has been co-published simultaneously as *Physical & Occupational Therapy in Pediatrics*, Volume 18, Number 1 1998.

The development, preparation, and publication of this work has been undertaken with great care. However, the publisher, employees, editors, and agents of The Haworth Press and all imprints of The Haworth Press, Inc., including The Haworth Medical Press® and Pharmaceutical Products Press®, are not responsible for any errors contained herein or for consequences that may ensue from use of materials or information contained in this work. Opinions expressed by the author(s) are not necessarily those of The Haworth Press, Inc.

First published by

The Haworth Press, Inc., 10 Alice Street, Binghamton, NY 13904-1580 USA

This edition published 2014 by Routledg
711 Third Avenue, New York, NY 10017
2 Park Square, Milton Park, Abingdon, Oxfordshire OX14 4RN

First issued in paperback 2014

Routledge is an imprint of the Taylor & Francis Group, an informa business

Cover design by Thomas J. Mayshock Jr.

Library of Congress Cataloging-in-Publication Data

Family-centred assessment and intervention in pediatric rehabilitation / Mary Law, editor.
        p. cm.
        "Has been co-published simultaneously as Physical & occupational therapy in pediatrics, volume 18, number 1 1998."
        Includes bibliographical references and index.
        ISBN 0-7890-0539-5 (alk. paper)
        1. Handicapped children–Rehabilitation. 2. Family services. 3. Handicapped children–Family relationships. I. Law, Mary C. II. Physical & occupational therapy in pediatrics.
RJ138.F36 1998
618.92'003–dc21   98-23945
                                                                                                  CIP

ISBN 13: 978-0-7890-0539-7 (hbk)
ISBN 13: 978-1-138-00238-8 (pbk)

Family-Centred Assessment and Intervention in Pediatric Rehabilitation

CONTENTS

ABOUT THE EDITOR

Mary Law, PhD, OT(C), is Associate Professor in the School of Rehabilitation Science and the Department of Clinical Epidemiology and Biostatistics at McMaster University in Ontario, Canada. She is also Director of the Neurodevelopmental Clinical Research Unit, a partnership between researchers at the University and 19 children's rehabilitation centres throughout Ontario. In addition, Dr. Law is a member of the American Academy of Cerebral Palsy and Developmental Medicine, the Academy of Research of the American Occupational Therapy Foundation, and the Canadian Association of Occupational Therapists. Her current interests include evaluating effectiveness of a family-centred intervention, continuing validation of the Canadian Occupational Performance Measure, and examining the environmental constraints which prohibit children with disabilities from participating in everyday activities.

ABOUT THE EDITOR

Family-Centred Service:
A Conceptual Framework
and Research Review

Peter Rosenbaum
Susanne King
Mary Law
Gillian King
Jan Evans

SUMMARY. Family-centred service (FCS) is a popular phrase widely used to encompass a set of ideas about service delivery to children
and their families. Despite the increasing adoption of the concepts of
FCS, however, many clinicians may remain uncertain about exactly
what FCS means. This review article has four purposes. The first
section presents a brief review of the history and ideas behind FCS.
Second, the authors present a new framework of FCS, blending the
elements of this approach into a set of ideas that have immediate
clinical applicability. The third focus of this paper is to review the

Peter Rosenbaum, MD, FRCP(C), is Developmental Pediatrician, Neurodevelopmental Clinical Research Unit (NCRU) Investigator, and Professor, Department of
Pediatrics, McMaster University, Hamilton, ON. Susanne King, MSc, is Research
Coordinator, NCRU. Mary Law, PhD, OT(C), is Director, NCRU, Associate Professor, School of Rehabilitation Science, McMaster University, Hamilton, and an occupational therapist. Gillian King, PhD, is NCRU Investigator, McMaster University,
Hamilton, and Research Director, Thames Valley Children's Centre (TVCC), London, ON. Jan Evans, MSc, is Physical Therapist, School Age and Adolescent Services Program, TVCC.

Address correspondence to: Peter Rosenbaum, NCRU, McMaster University,
Faculty of Health Sciences, T-16, Room 126, 1280 Main Street West, Hamilton,
ON, Canada L8S 4K1.

[Haworth co-indexing entry note]: "Family-Centred Service: A Conceptual Framework and Research
Review." Rosenbaum, Peter et al. Co-published simultaneously in *Physical & Occupational Therapy in
Pediatrics* (The Haworth Press, Inc.) Vol. 18, No. 1, 1998, pp. 1-20; and: *Family-Centred Assessment and
Intervention in Pediatric Rehabilitation* (ed: Mary Law) The Haworth Press, Inc., 1998, pp. 1-20. Single
or multiple copies of this article are available for a fee from The Haworth Document Delivery Service
[1-800-342-9678, 9:00 a.m. - 5:00 p.m. (EST). E-mail address: getinfo@haworthpressinc.com].

research evidence that supports FCS and to point to areas where further research is needed. Finally we consider the implications for service providers of the move to FCS, and the potential uses of the FCS framework as a guide for teaching and research. *[Article copies available for a fee from The Haworth Document Delivery Service: 1-800-342-9678. E-mail address: getinfo@haworthpressinc.com]*

INTRODUCTION

Jeremy is a bright four-year-old boy with dystonic cerebral palsy who communicates by making guttural noises but has no speech. He has had more than two years of speech therapy at the local treatment centre. His parents have been advised by the treatment centre staff that a program of sign language would be beneficial, because it would enable Jeremy to put his ideas across, albeit in an alternative mode of communication. His grandparents are very much against this approach, believing that if this is done Jeremy will be stigmatized and never learn to talk. Because the grandparents care for Jeremy after daycare, and sometimes on weekends while his parents work, Jeremy's parents are reluctant to go against their wishes. The parents come to discuss this dilemma with you.

This scenario could be reproduced in many variations to reflect contemporary issues in the delivery of child health services. Situations like these are indicative of an increasing expectation on the part of parents to be involved in and control decision-making in matters that concern themselves and their children. No longer can health professionals simply prescribe to parents in a top-down paternalistic model of care, with the beliefs that parents want to be told what to do and that they will actually do it. Equally it is no longer possible to disregard the wishes and hopes of parents about the things that are done for their children.

How should service providers respond to this expectation for parent involvement and control in issues of child health, especially in the context of chronic care? What models of service delivery are appropriate for these changing times, and what are the implications of these models for clinical practice? To a large extent the answers to questions like these lie in an understanding and adoption of the concepts subsumed under the broad umbrella of "Family-Centred Service."

The purpose of this article is to describe a framework of family-centred service (FCS) that addresses these issues. Building on elements of FCS that can be found in the literature, we set out to accomplish four goals: (a) to review briefly the history and ideas behind FCS; (b) to blend the elements of FCS into a conceptual framework; (c) to review research evidence that supports aspects of the framework (and points out gaps in our understanding and information); and (d) to consider the implications of FCS for service providers, addressing expectations concerning our attitudes and behaviours implicit in the contemporary practice of FCS.

BACKGROUND AND HISTORY OF FAMILY-CENTRED SERVICE

The nature of services to children with disabilities, and of the parent-professional relationship, has changed dramatically over the past 50 years.[1] During the first half of this century parents were viewed as incapable of raising their children with disabilities and thus institutional placement was recommended. In the 1940s and 1950s parents began to band together into advocacy groups. This began a slow evolution and shift away from professionals controlling the destiny of children with special needs to parents controlling the process in partnership with professionals. Many widespread social and political influences have converged to bring about these changes, of which the primary forces came from legislation, parental advocacy and current views of "best practice."[2]

Ideas about "client-centred" or "family-centred" practice originated in the 1940s with Carl Rogers' approach to working with families of problem children.[3] In the mid-1960s the Association for the Care of Children in Hospital (ACCH–now the Association for the Care of Children's Health) was founded and began to provide ideas about family-centred care. In the intervening 30 years, many organizations and authors have proposed concepts and discussed ways in which care and services should be offered to families of children with special health needs. To a great extent this literature is characterized by wisdom and insight, and is generally helpful in presenting the concepts behind the shift from authoritarian to partnership practice.

Intervention for children with chronic health problems or developmental disabilities has typically been child-centred with doctors and therapists setting goals which focus on bringing about changes in the child. The medical model of intervention views the health professional as the expert. The professional is able to assess the problems, recommend interventions, and provide or co-ordinate treatment. Over the past ten years the role of the family in the child's life has received increased recognition. Both research and parent advocacy have led health care professionals to a realization that parents have tremendous insights into their child's abilities and are valuable resources in their lives. Family systems theory emphasizes the interactions of various members of the family and the impact of each member upon all the others. This theory also proposes that when family members are physically and psychologically healthy they are more capable of facilitating their child's development.[4] This has led to the view that interventions can affect children indirectly by influencing other components of the family system.

The efforts of parent advocacy groups stimulated legislative changes in the United States that led to the enactment of the Education of All Handicapped Children Act in 1975, requiring parental involvement in decision-making about services for their children. Public Law 94-142 also mandated that parents be involved in setting goals and planning services for their children, which led to the development of an individual education plan.

Over the years parents have become knowledgeable consumers and now speak out actively about the types of services they require and how they want to be involved in the process of defining these services.[5] The research and personal experiences of parents such as the Turnbulls[6] have helped to sensitize service providers to the complexities of living with a child with a disability, and the needs of all the family members. Legislative revisions have been made to reflect these concerns, for example with PL 99-457 enacted in 1986, requiring that the total family be the recipients of services, and that the family members decide how they want to be involved in the decision-making process concerning goals and services for their child. Despite a growing body of literature outlining the processes of service provision, what has been less evident is a conceptual framework within which to place the many important ideas that flow from a belief in "family-centred" service.

CONCEPTUAL FRAMEWORK FOR FAMILY-CENTRED SERVICE

The Neurodevelopmental Clinical Research Unit (NCRU) at McMaster University is a multidisciplinary clinical research group working in partnership with all 19 of Ontario children's rehabilitation centres. In response to requests from our partner agencies to help conceptualize, teach and implement FCS, we reviewed the existing descriptive and research literatures on FCS (see Appendix A for a bibliography of this descriptive literature). We have attempted to distil the wisdom from this literature into a conceptual framework directed particularly to service providers and supported wherever possible by research evidence. (In addition we have undertaken studies to assess the degree of family-centredness of our partner agencies, as perceived both by parents and by professionals, the results of which are presented elsewhere.[7])

Family-centred service has been well defined by the National Center for Family-Centered Care as follows:

Family-centered *service* is the name that has been given to a constellation of new philosophies, attitudes, and approaches to care for children with special health service needs. At the very heart of family-centered *service* is the recognition that the family is the constant in a child's life. For this reason, family-centered *service* is built on partnerships between parents and professionals.[8] (We have altered the quotation from family-centered care to family-centered *service*.)

In practical terms, what does this statement mean, and more specifically, what are the implications for service providers? The NCRU's ideas about FCS (Table 1) are built upon a three-level framework that attempts to incorporate current ideas about FCS, and to offer both parent and professional perspectives on the issues. First, and central to the framework, are three basic premises or assumptions, consistently articulated in the literature as the backbone of FCS. Each assumption is followed by a small number of guiding principles or "should" statements, directed to service providers as the foundation upon which our interactions with families should be grounded. These are the logical consequences of each basic assumption. Note that the premises in this approach focus primarily on the family, while the guiding principles begin to describe the climate within which the parent-professional interaction "should" take place.

The third component of the framework, and what distinguishes this approach from many other conceptualizations of FCS,[9] is a series of "elements"–key service provider behaviours–that follow from the assumptions about families and the guiding principles with which they are associated. Note that these elements are all found in the literature and are not the creation of the present authors. We have simply tried to collect together those aspects of the philosophy and practice of FCS as they concern service providers, in a manner complementary to the parent-focused dimensions of the FCS model, and to make FCS more accessible and practicable to service providers. We also believe that an approach like this one makes it possible to identify how to both teach and measure FCS in practice.

The first basic premise of this model of FCS is that "Parents know their children best and want the best for their children." For service providers this means encouraging parental decision-making based upon appropriately presented information, in the context of clearly defined child and family needs, and built upon child and family strengths. The milieu in which such care and services are offered must be a collaborative partnership, with service providers as technical experts with knowledge and perspectives on the condition and treatments, and parents as experts on their child, their family, and their strengths, needs and values. Services should be offered in an accessible manner, both with respect to the location of the services and

TABLE 1. Premises, Principles, and Elements of Family-Centred Service

Premises (basic assumptions)	
• Parents know their children best and want the best for their children.	• Families are different and unique.
	• Optimal child functioning occurs within a supportive family and community context: The child is affected by the stress and coping of other family members.

Guiding Principles ("should" statements)	
• Each family should have the opportunity to decide the level of involvement they wish in decision-making for their child.	• Each family and family member should be treated with respect (as individuals).
• Parents should have ultimate responsibility for the care of their children.	• The needs of all family members should be considered.
	• The involvement of all family members should be supported and encouraged.

Elements (key service provider behaviours)		
Service Provider Behaviours	**Service Provider Behaviours**	**Service Provider Behaviours**
• to encourage parent decision-making	• to respect families	• to consider psychosocial needs of all members
• to assist in identifying strengths	• to support families	• to encourage participation of all members
• to provide information	• to listen	• to respect coping styles
• to assist in identifying needs	• to provide individualized service	• to encourage use of community supports
• to collaborate with parents	• to accept diversity	• to build on strengths
• to provide accessible services	• to believe and trust parents	
• to share information about the child	• to communicate clearly	

in a style that respects each family's abilities to understand and absorb information and advice. Obviously counselling must be based upon a clear and shared understanding of each child's situation.

The second premise of the NCRU framework posits that "Families are different and unique," and argues for the individualization of our services for each family and its members. The immediate implications for service providers include the need to recognize and accept the diversity of parental values and cultures found within our multi-ethnic communities. This premise demands that wherever possible we tailor our communications–both the facts and the examples we use–to be consistent with the individual understanding and needs of the families with whom we work. To identify parents as "typical" of this or that is not appropriate. Rather, we must strive to understand their predicaments in their terms, and advise them in their "language." Other fundamental elements of this approach include the ability to listen carefully to what parents are saying and to trust their observations about their child.

Pediatrics can be considered as a specialized form of family practice, because the ecological context of children is their family, within their community. The third premise of the FCS framework presented here reflects this reality of childhood, and states "Optimal child functioning occurs within a supportive family and community context: the child is affected by the stress and coping of other family members." If services for children with special health or developmental problems are to be family-centred, the needs and involvement of all family members should be encouraged and supported.

For service providers trained at, and practicing within, specialized hospital-based programs, this third notion of FCS may pose particular challenges. The need here is to look outward–toward the child's family and its needs; toward the involvement of family members (for example, grandparents) in the care of the child; to the use of community services and supports as valuable contributors to child and family well-being. This premise also challenges service providers to recognize and build upon each family's strengths, in the context of their individual coping styles, without judgments about those adaptations.

RESEARCH EVIDENCE IN SUPPORT OF FAMILY-CENTRED SERVICE

Any innovative treatment, intervention, or service delivery model requires both a theoretical and a scientific basis. Much has been written and discussed about the meaning of family-centred service and its purported benefits, which for many people intuitively have credibility. Prior to implementing changes in clinical and administrative practices, however, considering whether any research evidence supports the effectiveness of family-centred service is essential.

Literature Review. The first step in preparing to conduct a literature search on this topic was to clarify what kind of impact or effect to examine. If one assumes that the purpose of working with families who have a child with a disability is to enhance the quality of life for that child and the family,[10] then the outcomes of interest for a family-centred framework should focus on more than the child's physical, emotional, social, and cognitive functioning. Within the ecological context of the child's development,[11] outcomes related to parents, siblings, the family unit, parent-child interactions, parent-professional relationships, health care providers, and the community would also have relevance in demonstrating the benefits of family-centred service.[12-15]

The literature search examined multiple databases (Medline, PsychInfo, Cumulative Index to Nursing and Allied Health Literature {CINAHL}, and Health Planning and Administration). The inconsistencies of terminology limited the search to several synonyms of "family- or patient- or client-centred" but individual features of a family-centred approach were not specifically searched for at this time. Few studies addressed the effectiveness of family-centred service in pediatric populations.

Organization and Presentation of Research Studies. The studies that were examined for evidence of the effectiveness of family-centred service were classified by the type of research design used. Four such classes are identified.[16] Class 4 evidence is the weakest and refers to descriptive and case studies and expert opinion. Cross-sectional and case-control studies provide Class 3 evidence. Class 2 evidence is derived from non-randomized controlled trials and before-after studies where subjects act as their own controls but no other control group exists. Class 1 evidence is obtained from randomized controlled trials and is the most powerful method available for evaluating effectiveness because of its features of a concurrent control group, random allocation of subjects by the investigator, balance of known and unknown confounders, and prospective data collection. Space permits only discussion of Class 1 evidence; however studies in Classes 2-4[17-27] are referenced in Tables 2 and 3, summarizing how all the available studies relate to the FCS framework.

Five Class 1 studies were found in the pediatric literature that are noteworthy. Moxley-Haegert and Serbin[28] randomly assigned 39 parents to one of three groups in a study to assess whether teaching parents to recognize developmental gains in their delayed infants would increase parents' participation in a home treatment program and thus enhance their

TABLE 2. Notation of References to Research Evidence Supporting the Effectiveness of Family-Centred Service Elements

Premises (basic assumptions)		
• Parents know their children best and want the best for their children.	• Families are different and unique.	• Optimal child functioning occurs within a supportive family and community context: The child is affected by the stress and coping of other family members.

Guiding Principles ("should" statements)		
• Each family should have the opportunity to decide the level of involvement they wish in decision-making for their child. • Parents should have ultimate responsibility for the care of their children.	• Each family and family member should be treated with respect (as individuals).	• The needs of all family members should be considered. • The involvement of all family members should be supported and encouraged.

Elements (key service provider behaviours)		
Service Provider Behaviours	**Service Provider Behaviours**	**Service Provider Behaviours**
• to encourage parent decision-making[17,18,26,31] • to assist in identifying strengths[17,18,25,26,28-31] • to provide information[20,22,23,25,26,28,29] • to assist in identifying needs[18,23,25,26,30,31] • to collaborate with parents[17,18,25,26] • to provide accessible services[19,25] • to share information about the child[20,28,29,31]	• to respect families[21,23,24,26] • to support families[17] • to listen[17,20,24] • to provide individualized service[25,26,28-31] • to accept diversity[26] • to believe and trust parents • to communicate clearly	• to consider psychosocial needs of all members[25,26,31] • to encourage participation of all members[26] • to respect coping styles • to encourage use of community supports • to build on strengths

TABLE 3. Research Evidence on Family-Centred Service: Summary of Outcome Measures Used in These Studies

CLASS 4 EVIDENCE	CLASS 3 EVIDENCE	CLASS 2 EVIDENCE	CLASS 1 EVIDENCE

1. Dunst et al.[21]
  • sense of control
	1-3. Dunst et al.[20]
	  • self-efficacy
	
	4. Brinker et al.[18]
	  • stress
	
	5. Korsch et al.[22]
	  • satisfaction
	
	6. Lewis et al.[23]
	  • distress reduction
	
	7. Miller et al.[25]
	  • psychological distress
	
	8. Street[26]
	  • satisfaction
	
	9. Wasserman et al.[27]
	  • satisfaction
	  • decrease in concerns
	  • opinions about clinician
		1. Marcenko & Smith[24]
		  • access to services
		  • maternal life satisfaction
		
		2. Caro & Derevensky[19]
		  • rate of infants' developmental gains
		  • families' functional skills satisfaction
		  • child targeted goals
		  • family members' goals
			1. Moxley-Haegert & Serbin[28]
			  • child skills
			  • motor developmental gains
			  • parents' knowledge acquisition
			  • parents' participation in home treatment program
			  • parents' ability to discriminate & report gains
			
			2. Parker et al.[29]
			  • mental & motor developmental gains
			  • child temperament
			  • home environment
			
			3. Davis & Gettinger[30]
			  • parents' preferences about assessment method
			  • nature & amount of information from assessment
			  • parents' evaluation of assessment experience
			
			4. Stein & Jessop[31,32]
			  • satisfaction with care
			  • child psychological adjustment
			  • mother's psychiatric symptoms
			  • impact on family
			  • child functional status
			  • follow-up study on child's psychological adjustment
			
			5. Pless et al.[34]
			  • child behaviour problems
			  • child's psychosocial adjustment
			  • child's self-worth

child's development. The developmental education (DE) group, which received a brief course on child development from an educator who visited the home, was compared to a group receiving parent education in child management, and to a no-education control group. The authors reported several positive parent outcomes for the DE group in comparison with the other two groups: greater acquisition of developmental knowledge, increased participation in the home treatment program and continued involvement with that program at one-year follow-up, and greater ability to discriminate and report their infants' developmental gains. In comparing the groups on child outcomes, children in the DE group achieved more skills that were the target of the home program and had greater motor development gains. Other aspects of developmental progress did not differ among the three groups.

A randomized controlled study by Parker, Zahr, Cole, and Brecht[29] demonstrated that a similar developmental intervention in the neonatal intensive care unit for 41 mothers of preterm infants was effective. Infants in the experimental group showed mental and motor gains, their mothers rated their temperaments as less difficult, and the home environment was more developmentally appropriate. These two studies[28,29] demonstrated that an educational program that focused on the family-centred elements of providing general and specific information, building on parents' skills, and individualizing services resulted in more parental involvement and positive outcomes for both children and parents.

In a study by Davis and Gettinger[30] 43 parents of children with special needs were randomly assigned to one of three family-focused assessment methods: (1) self-report measures, (2) self-report measures combined with a structured interview, and (3) an open-ended interview. The purpose was to examine parents' preferences among assessment methods, the nature and amount of information obtained about a family, and parents' evaluations of their assessment experiences. At pre-assessment, more parents preferred the method of completing self-report measures along with a structured interview vs. either the self-report measures alone, or an interview. At post-assessment, however, all three methods were evaluated highly by parents regardless of whether they received their preferred method. Only minimal differences were found across methods in the nature and amount of information gathered about a family's strengths, resources, concerns, and priorities.

These data showed high evaluations across the assessment methods because each incorporated the family-centred elements of assisting families to identify their strengths and needs. Varying preferences for a particular method among families also emphasized the importance of individualizing services. These are important findings in themselves to support family-centred service; nevertheless, this study could have provided more definitive research evidence on the effectiveness of a family-centred approach if a control or comparison group that did not receive a family-focused assessment had been used.

The work by Stein and Jessop[31,32] offers additional support for several elements of the family-centred framework. In a randomized controlled trial, 219 families of children with chronic illness were assigned to receive either the Pediatric Home Care program (PHC) or standard care (SC) as the control condition.[31] The PHC was described as "an integrated biomedical and psychosocial approach" that focused on the whole family and its needs, while the standard care was comprised of those services traditionally offered at their hospital. Of the five outcomes assessed, two differed significantly between the PHC and SC groups, with the PHC group showing greater parental satisfaction with care and better psychological adjustment of the child. Mothers' psychiatric symptoms also lessened although this finding did not reach statistical significance. No differences between the groups were found on a measure of the impact of the child's condition on the family and on the child's functional status. In a follow-up study 4.5-5 years later, Stein and Jessop[32] demonstrated the long-term effects of the PHC program when the PHC children scored significantly better on overall adjustment and significantly higher on four of the six subscales of the Personal Adjustment and Role Skills scale,[33] the same measure used in their earlier work.

These positive results deserve further comment. The authors indicated that the PHC program encouraged families to become more actively involved in taking responsibility for managing their child's care and for making informed decisions in partnership with the health care providers. The PHC program also included coordinating services, health education, and support. Although its name indicates a home-based model of care delivery, services were provided in other traditional locations where appropriate such as clinics, in-patient units, the PHC office, school and community, thus demonstrating its individualized approach. Many of the features described here and in the above paragraph are the same elements outlined in the Family-Centred Service framework and are represented across all three premises of the framework.

Pless and colleagues[34] conducted a randomized controlled study to examine the effectiveness of a specialized nursing intervention in reducing or preventing adjustment problems in children with chronic physical disabilities. The nurses focused on overall concerns of the child *and* family, provided support and individualized services, and collaborated with the families to identify their needs and strengths, to build on the family's strengths, and to obtain the services families needed. Compared with the control group (n = 161), the children receiving the intervention (n – 171) were significantly different on two of the three outcome measures. These children had higher scores compared with controls on a parent-completed measure of function and role performance, indicating better psychosocial adjustment, and had significantly better scores on several subscales of a child measure of self-worth. The groups did not differ on a measure of child behaviour problems. Their findings support the effectiveness of a family-centred approach, in this case as offered by nurses, to help reduce or prevent children's adjustment problems.

Summary of Research Evidence. This review of pediatric research demonstrates considerable evidence of the effectiveness of a family-centred approach to service delivery. Sixteen of the 19 elements in the Family-Centred Service framework have been addressed in studies of varying quality (Table 2). Research using all classes of evidence has been directed at every element under the first premise. Under the second premise, the elements of "respect families," "provide individualized care," and "accept diversity" are supported by rigorous evidence. Unfortunately, the elements of "support families" and "listen" have received little attention while "believe and trust parents" and "communicate clearly" were not identified specifically in any of the studies. Some elements under the third premise have been examined by several researchers using Class 1 or 2 evidence. Although the element, "encourage use of community supports," has been studied only minimally, the research evidence as cited by Shelton[35] on the benefit and effectiveness of family and parent support programs is why service providers are *encouraged* to do those things that make a difference. The other two elements under the third premise have received little or no attention.

Another way of summarizing these findings is to identify what outcomes have and have not been examined. Table 3 outlines the outcomes used in the studies reviewed in this section. Satisfaction is an outcome in many of the studies and is represented across three of the four classes of evidence. The outcomes in Classes 3 and 4 focus on parent outcomes while those for the studies with stronger evidence of effectiveness under Classes 1 and 2 generally include child and family outcomes in addition to parent ones. Future research must continue to employ outcomes from multiple perspectives as well as to increase the breadth of outcomes studied.[35-37]

In addition to recognizing the need for further research on the less studied elements of the family-centred framework, and for the inclusion and expansion of the types of outcome measures used, other factors need consideration in making sense of these studies and their results. As indicated at the beginning of this research evidence section, this review may not include relevant studies due partly to the varying terminology, and the multi-dimensional nature of this framework. This problem is highlighted by the Caro and Derevensky[19] (a Class 2 study) and the Stein and Jessop[31] studies which examined an entire program of service delivery. These authors could not discern which elements, acting either alone or in some combination with other elements, produced the positive results. No negative findings were included in this review because none were found; however, this may be due to biases against investigating, reporting or publishing negative results.

The findings presented in this review provide considerable support for the effectiveness of family-centred service, and point to future research directions. The evidence presented here must be built upon by continuing to search in the literature for well-designed studies that target, in particular, those elements outlined above that have received little or no research attention. The findings need to be replicated, and longitudinal studies are needed to examine the long-term effectiveness of a family-centred approach to service delivery. As well, cost-benefit analyses should be incorporated into research studies to assist practice and policy decision-making.[38]

IMPLICATIONS OF FCS FOR SERVICE PROVIDERS

Ultimately whether one adopts this particular framework of FCS or another, it is clear that service provision for children with chronic problems of health or development will continue to evolve in the direction of parent and family control of what is done.[39] This notion can be both liberating and threatening for service providers.

The threats are apparent. Service providers are no longer revered as authorities to whom parents turn uncritically for wisdom and advice. Professionals are being recognized as human and fallible, and even when our advice is sound people may not wish to listen to our formulations! This shift in power relationships can easily lead service providers to feel devalued, unskilled and puzzled by the changes from roles we have traditionally adopted. Some people may wish to cling to the old models, in the hope that this trend will vanish. At times parents may make choices that are different from what we believe are the "best" decisions. They do so by weighing up factors that may include our advice, but likely incorporate other considerations unknown to us. These actions and judgments are the parents' responsibility, and unless they make decisions that put a child at physical or psychological risk, parents have to be respected.

On the other hand, in an era of FCS the responsibilities for the well-being of children have shifted back where they belong (and in fact always were)–to the family. Service providers are no longer bearing the burden of curing and caring, as might have been the case at a time when paternalistic health care was the prevalent model. Rather, parents now seek partnerships with service providers built on trust, respect, enablement and acceptance of them as competent individuals. Service providers continue to be consulted for their knowledge and perspectives, and parents want their ideas about diagnosis, prognosis and management. Nevertheless, the interpersonal dimensions of FCS–the "elements" in the model of FCS presented here–are the aspects of care and services to which service providers in the 90s must address themselves. Parents have access to enormous amounts of information and often know more facts about the child's condition than we. Still research by our group[40] and others[41,42] indicates that parents continue to report that, in general, their needs for information are not being met adequately. In addition, what they want from service providers are the elements of caring and support that cannot be found in books or on the Internet.

The skeptic may feel that all these FCS ideas are mere words for things they have always known and done anyway. Because these ideas represent a shift rather than a radical departure into totally new realms of practice, they can in some ways be harder to adopt than a totally novel approach. The experience of our research group in helping others understand and implement this FCS framework has been that adoption is a process rather than an endpoint. We believe that people who are honest, prepared to reflect on their beliefs and values, and open to considering the perspectives of others (particularly parents) will find the challenges well worth the work required to adapt, and to adopt FCS ideas.

The FCS framework presented here appears to have value as a teaching tool. Furthermore adoption of a model of FCS such as this framework also provides service providers or programs with a basis on which to measure both the perceptions of parents and their own behaviours. Several investigators[40,43,44] have created instruments to evaluate the degree of family-centredness of programs from both parental and service provider perspectives. We believe that such program evaluation will become increasingly important as expectations for family-centred services grow.

Returning briefly to the case scenario that opened this paper, how might one use the concepts of FCS to address parental concerns and the dilemmas of the service providers? Jeremy's parents are clearly caught in a difficult bind, wanting to listen to their professional advisors, but not wanting to disagree with Jeremy's grandparents. In a situation like this the service providers might suggest a joint visit with the grandparents–perhaps at the family's home–in order for everyone to explore the issues together. Such an approach respects the family's need to be in charge, accepts the reality of the extended family's role in influencing decision-making, and brings the professional perspectives to the family in a way which respects their integrity. The family could be offered the chance to meet and talk with other parents who have been in the same dilemma as they now face, and to learn how they have made their decisions. If the parents still do not want to implement an alternative communication system, the service providers working with Jeremy and his family should respect that decision; however, they might also find it useful to set some specific behavioural goals for Jeremy, and a time-line by which these will be evaluated and the present decisions reviewed. By doing this they would be demonstrating acceptance of the parents' choice; at the same time they would have negotiated a plan that might be acceptable to all concerned. The mere act of respecting and supporting the parental dilemma might ease the parents' mind, increase their trust in Jeremy's service providers, and make their next encounter more comfortable and productive for everyone.

REFERENCES

1. Leviton A, Mueller M, Kauffman C. The family-centered consultation model: practical applications for professionals. *Inf Young Children*. 1992;4(3):1-8.

2. Bailey DB, Buysse V, Edmondson R, Smith TM. Creating family-centred services in early intervention: perceptions of professionals in four states. *Except Child*. 1992;58:298-309.

3. Rogers CR. *Client-centered Therapy*. Boston, MA: Houghton-Mifflin; 1951.

4. Odom SL, Yoder P, Hill G. Developmental intervention for infants with handicaps: purposes and programs. *J Spec Ed*. 1988;22:11-24.

5. Simeonson RJ, Bailey DB. Family dimensions in early intervention. In: Meisels SJ, Shonkoff JP, eds. *Handbook of Early Childhood Intervention*. New York, NY: Cambridge University Press; 1990.

6. Turnbull HR, Turnbull AP. *Parents Speak Out Then and Now*. 2nd ed. Columbus, OH: Charles E. Merrill; 1985.

7. King G, Law M, King S, Rosenbaum P. Parents' and service providers' perceptions of the family-centredness of children's rehabilitation services in Ontario. *Phys Occup Ther Pediatr*. 1998;18(1):21-40.

8. National Center for Family-Centered Care. *What Is Family-Centered Care?* (brochure) Bethesda, MD: Association for the Care of Children's Health; 1990.

9. Shelton TL, Stepanek JS. *Family-Centered Care for Children Needing Specialized Health and Development Services.* 3rd ed. Bethesda, MD: Association for the Care of Children's Health; 1994.

10. Fewell RR, Vadasy PF. Measurement issues in studies of efficacy. *Top Early Child Spec Educ.* 1987;7(2):85-96.

11. Bronfenbrenner V. Toward an experimental ecology of human development. *Am Psychol.* 1977;32:513-531.

12. Allen DA. Measuring rehabilitation outcomes for infants and young children. In: Fuhrer MJ, ed. *Rehabilitation Outcomes Analysis and Measurement.* Baltimore, MD: Paul H. Brookes; 1987:185-195.

13. Bennett FC, Guralnick MJ. Effectiveness of developmental intervention in the first five years of life. *Pediatr Clin North Am.* 1991;38:1513-1528.

14. Epstein SG, Taylor AB, Halberg AS, Gardner JD, Klein Walker D, Crocker AC. *Enhancing Quality—Standards and Indicators of Quality Care for Children with Special Health Care Needs.* Boston, MA: New England SERVE; 1989.

15. Simeonsson RJ. Evaluating the effects of family-focused intervention. In: Bailey DB Jr, Simeonsson RJ, eds. *Family Assessment in Early Intervention.* Columbus. OH: Merrill; 1988:251-267.

16. Sackett DL, Haynes RB, Guyatt GH, Tugwell P. *Clinical Epidemiology. A Basic Science for Clinical Medicine.* 2nd ed. Boston, MA: Little, Brown; 1991.

17. Bailey DB, Simeonson RJ, Winton PJ, Huntington GS, Comfort M, Isbell P, O'Donnell KJ, Helm JM. Family-focused intervention: a functional model for planning, implementing, and evaluating individualized family services in early intervention. *J Div Early Child.* 1986;10:156-171.

18. Brinker RP, Seifer R, Sameroff AJ. Relations among maternal stress, cognitive development, and early intervention in middle- and low-SES infants with developmental disabilities. *Am J Ment Retard.* 1994;98(4):463-480.

19. Caro P, Derevensky JL. Family-focused intervention model: implementation and research findings. *Top Early Child Spec Educ.* 1991;11(3):66-80.

20. Dunst CJ, Trivette CM, Boyd K, Brookfield J. Helpgiving practices and the self-efficacy appraisals of parents. In: Dunst CJ, Trivette CM, Deal AG, eds. *Supporting and Strengthening Families (Vol. 1): Methods, Strategies and Practices.* Cambridge, MA: Brookline Books; 1994:212-220.

21. Dunst CJ, Trivette CM, Davis M, Cornwall J. Enabling and empowering families of children with health impairments. *Child Health Care.* 1988;17:71-81.

22. Korsch BM, Gozzi EK, Francis V. Gaps in doctor-patient communication: I. Doctor-patient interaction and patient satisfaction. *Pediatrics.* 1968;42:855-871.

23. Lewis CC, Scott DE, Pantell RH, Wolf MH. Parent satisfaction with children's medical care. Development, field test, and validation of a questionnaire. *Med Care.* 1986;24:209-215.

24. Marcenko MO, Smith LK. The impact of a family-centered case management approach. *Social Work in Health Care.* 1992;17(1):87-100.

25. Miller AC, Gordon RM, Daniele RJ, Diller L. Stress, appraisal, and coping in mothers of disabled and nondisabled children. *J Pediatr Psychol.* 1992; 17(5): 587-605.

26. Street RL. Physicians' communication and parents' evaluations of pediatric consultations. *Med Care.* 1991;29:1146-1152.

27. Wasserman RC, Inui TS, Barriatua RD, Carter WB, Lippincott P. Pediatric clinicians' support for parents makes a difference: an outcome-based analysis of clinician-parent interaction. *Pediatrics.* 1984;74:1047-1053.

28. Moxley-Haegert L, Serbin LA. Developmental education for parents of delayed infants: effects on parental motivation and children's development. *Child Dev.* 1983;54:1324-1331.

29. Parker SJ, Zahr LK, Cole JG, Brecht M-L. Outcome after developmental intervention in the neonatal intensive care unit for mothers of preterm infants with low socioeconomic status. *J Pediatr.* 1992;120:780-785.

30. Davis SK, Gettinger M. Family-focused assessment for identifying family resources and concerns: parent preferences, assessment information, and evaluation across three methods. *J Sch Psychol.* 1995;33:99-121.

31. Stein REK, Jessop DJ. Does pediatric home care make a difference for children with chronic illness? Findings from the pediatric ambulatory care treatment study. *Pediatrics.* 1984;73:845-853.

32. Stein REK, Jessop DJ. Long-term mental health effects of a pediatric home care program. *Pediatrics.* 1991;88:490-496.

33. Ellsworth R, Ellsworth S. CAAP Scale: The Measurement of Child and Adolescent Adjustment. Palo Alto, CA: Consulting Psychologists Press; 1982.

34. Pless IB, Feeley N, Gottlieb L, Rowat K, Daugherty G, Willard B. Randomized trial of a nursing intervention to promote the adjustment of children with chronic physical disabilities. *Pediatrics.* 1994;94:70-75.

35. Shelton TL. Family-centered care: does it work? In: Hostler S, ed. *Family-Centered Care: An Approach to Implementation.* Charlottesville, VA: University of Virginia; 1994:411-453.

36. O'Brien M, Dale D. Family-centered services in the neonatal intensive care unit: a review of research. *J Early Interv.* 1994;18(1):78-90.

37. Shonkoff JP, Hauser-Cram P, Kraus MW, Upshur CC. Early intervention efficacy research: what have we learned and where do we go from here? *Top Early Child Spec Educ.* 1988;8(1):81-93.

38. Barnett WS, Escobar CM. Economic costs and benefits of early intervention. In: Meisels SJ, Shonkoff JP, eds. *Handbook of Early Childhood Intervention.* Cambridge, MA: Cambridge University Press; 1990:560-582.

39. Trivette CM, Dunst CJ, Allen S, Wall L. Family-centeredness of the Children's Health Care journal. *Child Health Care.* 1993;22(4):241-256.

40. King SM, Rosenbaum PL, King G. Parents' perceptions of care-giving: development and validation of a measure of processes. *Dev Med Child Neurol.* 1996;38:757-772.

41. Cleary PD, Edgman-Levitan S, Roberts M, Moloney TW, McMullen W, Walker JD, Delbanco TL. Patients evaluate their hospital care: a national survey. *Health Affairs.* 1991;Winter.

42. von Essen L, Sjödén P. Perceived occurrence and importance of caring behaviours among patients and staff in psychiatric, medical and surgical care. *J Adv Nurs.* 1995;21:266-276.

43. Murphy D, Lee I. *Family-Centered Program Rating Scale User's Manual.* 2nd ed. Lawrence, KS: The University of Kansas, Beach Center on Families and Disability; 1991.

44. Rosenbaum P, King S, King G. The measure of processes of care–service provider version (MPOC-SP): preliminary data. (Unpublished observations).

APPENDIX A

Sources of Information for the Family-Centred Service Framework

Beach Center on Families and Disability. Quality criteria for family support programs. *Beach Center on Families and Disability Newsletter;* 1993

Boumbulian PJ, MacGregor WD, Delbanco TL, Edgman-Levitan S, Smith DR, Anderson RJ. Patient-centered patient-valued care. *J Health Care Poor Underserved.* 1991;2:338-346

Brewer EJ Jr, McPherson M, Magrab PR, Hutchins VL. Family-centered, community-based, coordinated care for children with special health care needs. *Pediatrics.* 1989;83:1055-1060

Dunst C, Trivette C, Deal A. *Enabling and Empowering Families.* Cambridge, MA: Brookline Books; 1988

Dunst C, Trivette C. An enablement and empowerment perspective of case management. *Top Early Child Spec Educ.* 1989;8:87-100

Epstein SG, Taylor AB, Halberg AS, Gardner JD, Klein Walker D, Crocker AC. *Enhancing Quality–Standards and Indicators of Quality Care for Children with Special Health Care Needs.* Boston, MA: New England SERVE; 1989

Johns N, Harvey C. Training for work with parents: strategies for engaging practitioners who are uninterested or resistant. *Inf Young Children.* 1993;5(4):52-57

McInnes S, Spence J. Family-centered care: our vision for the future. *Workshop presented at The Children's Rehabilitation Centre of Essex County.* Windsor, ON; 1993

Murphy D, Lee I. *Family-Centered Program Rating Scale User's Manual.* 2nd ed. Lawrence, KS: The University of Kansas, Beach Center on Families and Disability; 1991

National Center for Family-Centered Care. *What Is Family-Centered*

Care? (brochure) Bethesda, MD: Association for the Care of Children's Health; 1990

Roberts RN, Magrab PR. Psychologists' role in a family-centered approach to practice, training, and research with young children. *Am Psychol.* 1991;46:144-148

Shelton TL, Jeppson ES, Johnson BH. *Family-Centered Care for Children with Special Health Care Needs.* 2nd ed. Washington, DC: Association for the Care of Children's Health; 1989

Summers JA. Family-Friendly Strategies for Gathering Information on Family Strengths and Needs. Preconference training workshop conducted at the Sixth International Early Childhood Conference on Children with Special Needs, International Division for Early Childhood of the Council for Exceptional Children, Albuquerque, NM; 1990

Trivette CM, Dunst CJ, Allen S, Wall L. Family-centeredness of the Children's Health Care journal. *Child Health Care.* 1993;22:241-256

Tunali B, Power TG. Creating satisfaction: a psychological perspective on stress and coping in families of handicapped children. *J Child Psychol Psychiatry.* 1993;34:945-957

Wertlieb D. Special section editorial: Toward a family centered pediatric psychology–challenge and opportunity in the International Year of the Family. *J Pediatr Psychol.* 1993;18:541-547

Parents' and Service Providers' Perceptions of the Family-Centredness of Children's Rehabilitation Services

Gillian King
Mary Law
Susanne King
Peter Rosenbaum

SUMMARY. Little is known about the extent to which children's re-habilitation services are delivered in a family-centred manner. In this article we report the results of two province-wide surveys, one con-

Gillian King, PhD, is Neurodevelopmental Clinical Research Unit (NCRU) Investigator, McMaster University, Hamilton, ON, and Research Director, Thames Valley Children's Centre, London, ON. Mary Law, PhD, OT(C), is Director, NCRU, Associate Professor, School of Rehabilitation Science, McMaster University and an occupational therapist. Susanne King, MSc, is Research Coordinator, NCRU. Peter Rosenbaum, MD, FRCP(C), is Developmental Pediatrician, NCRU Investigator and Professor, Department of Pediatrics, McMaster University.

Address correspondence to: Gillian King, PhD, Thames Valley Children's Centre, 779 Base Line Road East, London, ON, Canada N6C 5Y6.

The authors greatly appreciate the support of the Ontario Association of Children's Rehabilitation Services and of the many parents and service providers who assisted us with this research.

This research has been made possible through the authors membership in the Neurodevelopmental Clinical Research Unit, a health system-linked research unit funded by The Ontario Ministry of Health. The authors also wish to acknowledge The Ontario Mental Health Foundation and The Ontario Ministry of Health for research grant funding.

[Haworth co-indexing entry note]: "Parents' and Service Providers' Perceptions of the Family-Centredness of Children's Rehabilitation Services." King, Gillian et al. Co-published simultaneously in *Physical & Occupational Therapy in Pediatrics* (The Haworth Press, Inc.) Vol. 18, No. 1, 1998, pp. 21-40; and: *Family-Centred Assessment and Intervention in Pediatric Rehabilitation* (ed: Mary Law) The Haworth Press, Inc., 1998, pp. 21-40. Single or multiple copies of this article are available for a fee from The Haworth Document Delivery Service [1-800-342-9678, 9:00 a.m. - 5:00 p.m. (EST). E-mail address: getinfo@haworthpressinc.com].

ducted with 436 parents and the other with 309 service providers, in which we examined the level of family-centred service in children's rehabilitation centres in Ontario, Canada. In one survey we employed the Measure of Processes of Care (MPOC), a measure of parents' perceptions of the behaviours of service providers, and in the other we employed the Family-Centered Program Rating Scale (FamPRS), a measure of service providers' perceptions of the importance and occurrence of family-centred service. The results of the two surveys were very similar. The responses of both parents and service providers indicated that centres were doing well with respect to the interpersonal aspects of service delivery, but that the provision of information was a relatively weak area. The implications of the findings and the utility of the two measurement tools are discussed, as are directions for future research. *[Article copies available for a fee from The Haworth Document Delivery Service: 1-800-342-9678. E-mail address: getinfo@haworthpressinc.com]*

During the past 20 years, families of children with disabilities or chronic illnesses have increased their role in the determination and implementation of services for their children. Families have been leaders in promoting family-centred service, a philosophy of service provision that emphasizes their central role in making decisions about the care their children receive.[1] Although the term "client-centred practice" first originated with Carl Rogers'[2] book on clinical intervention with the problem child, use of the term "family-centred service" and the implementation of the principles of family-centred service has emerged only during the last ten years.[3] Challenged by changes in the health services field and increased demand by consumers for involvement in the services they receive, health care providers are beginning to define and implement family-centred service.

"Family-centred service" is a term which arose from early intervention programs in the United States. A number of important concepts define family-centred service, including the following principles: (a) Parents know their children best and want the best for their children; (b) Families are different and unique; and (c) Optimal child functioning occurs within a supportive family and community context: The child is affected by the stress and coping of other family members.[4]

In family-centred service, the right of each family to make autonomous decisions is a particular emphasis. The relationship between the family and professionals is a partnership in which the families define the priorities for intervention and, with the service provider, help to direct the intervention process.[5] In working with families, service providers emphasize parent education to enable parents to make informed choices about the therapeutic needs of their child.[6] Intervention is based on families' visions and values. Service providers recognize their own values and do not impose them on families. The families' roles, interests, the environments in which they live, and their culture are recognized as important in service provision.[7] Individualization of both the assessment and the intervention process is emphasized. Intervention is seen as a dynamic process in which clinicians and parents work together as partners to define the therapeutic needs of the child with a disability. Services are designed to fit the needs of families, rather than families fitting the services or interventions that are already in place.

The literature provides evidence that multidisciplinary, family-centred service for children with disabilities leads to increased family satisfaction and greater functional improvement in children with disabilities.[4] Research has demonstrated that parents felt increased control when service providers were positive and proactive, and promoted parental participation and competency.[5] Parents felt a lack of control when service providers were unresponsive to the family's needs, paternalistic, and failed to recognize or accept family decisions.[5] Moxley-Haegert and Serbin[8] found that teaching parents to recognize developmental gains in their delayed infants increased parents' participation and enhanced developmental gains for the children. Stein and Jessop,[9,10] in a randomized controlled trial with 219 families, demonstrated that an integrated, community-based program that focused on the whole family and its needs led to greater parental satisfaction with care and better psychological adjustment of the child.

The previously described literature indicates the importance of providing children's rehabilitation services in a family-centred manner, but what is the current level of family-centred service provided in children's rehabilitation centres? Do parents and service providers have similar perceptions of the extent of the occurrence of the different aspects of caregiving that make up family-centred service? This article addresses these issues.

Few large-scale surveys of patient-centred care or family-centred service have been published. The Picker-Commonwealth group[11] reported the results of a national telephone survey of 6,455 adult patients recently discharged from 62 hospitals in the United States. Their Picker-Commonwealth Survey of Patient-Centered Care examined five areas: patient education and communication with providers, respect for patients' needs and preferences, the provision of emotional and physical comfort, family involvement, and discharge preparation. The problems most frequently reported by patients included lack of information about the daily hospital routine (45%) and not having a relationship of trust with any hospital staff members other than the physician in charge of their care (39%).

In a recent Swedish study[12] the perceptions of 123 patients and 123 staff members with respect to the importance and occurrence of 50 caring behaviours were compared (using the CARE-Q and CARE-How often questionnaires). In psychiatric, medical, and surgical care, both staff and patients agreed fairly well in their rankings of the occurrence of the behaviours (although staff overestimated the occurrence of the behaviours in comparison to patients). Staff and patients did, however, differ in their rankings of the importance of the behaviours. Patients considered explanatory behaviours, the development of a trusting relationship, and monitoring and follow through to be more important than did staff members, whereas staff rated being accessible and comforting patients as more important. According to von Essen and Sjödén,[12] little attention has been paid to what patients perceive as caring behaviours, and comparisons between staff member and patient perceptions are even more scarce.

As part of an instrument development study, Mahoney, O'Sullivan, and Dennebaum[13] surveyed a national sample of 503 mothers to determine their perceptions of the family-centredness of early intervention programs. The children of these mothers had a wide variety of conditions, including Down Syndrome, cerebral palsy, and other medical conditions associated with mental retardation. Mothers reported "sometimes" receiving information about their child ($M = 4.4$ on a 6-point scale) but almost never receiving assistance directed at their well-being or that of other family members ($M = 2.6$).

No large-scale surveys have been conducted on the family-centredness of rehabilitation services for children with chronic conditions in Canada or the United States. In the present article we report data from two province-wide surveys that have provided information about the extent of family-centred services in children's rehabilitation centres in Ontario, Canada. One survey provided the perspective of parents and the other provided the perspective of staff members.

METHOD

Rehabilitation services for children with disabilities in the province of Ontario, Canada, are provided through 20 geographically-based children's centres, all but one of which provide ambulatory services. These centres provide a broad range of services to over 18,000 children within the province. Almost all children with disabilities in the province receive at least some (if not the majority) of their services from these centres. We conducted two surveys to examine the extent to which family-centred concepts were perceived to be present in the services provided by these centres. Both parents' and service providers' perceptions of services were the focus of this research.

The Measurement Tools

Measure of Processes of Care (MPOC). Parents' perceptions of the caregiving provided by the centres were obtained using the Measure of Processes of Care (MPOC).[14,15] MPOC was developed with extensive input from parents and is based on aspects of care that parents view as important.[16,17] Because the MPOC measures many of the concepts of family-centred service that are described in the literature (such as the extent to which parents are provided with information and encouraged to make decisions), it can be considered a measure of the extent to which services are family-centred.

The MPOC asks "to what extent" parents experience a variety of service provider behaviours that are important to parents of children with chronic health and development problems. Parents are asked to indicate "*how much* this event or situation happens to you" on a 7-point scale (1 = "never," 4 = "sometimes," and 7 = "to a great extent"). A "non-applicable" category is also included. Scale scores are calculated by averaging the scores of all items on a scale. No overall MPOC score is calculated. Through factor analysis, the original 101-item measure was refined to a 56-item questionnaire with five scales.

The five scales are described below. **Enabling and Partnership** (16 items) assesses parents' perceptions of their involvement in the care process. The scale includes behaviours such as providing parents with opportunities to make decisions about treatment, explaining treatment choices fully, and enabling parents to choose when to receive information and the type of information they would prefer. **Providing General Information** (9 items) focuses on activities that meet parents' general information needs. It includes behaviours such as providing information to parents, providing advice on how to get information, and providing information about services available in the community. **Providing Specific Information about the Child** (5 items) assesses behaviours by which parents are provided with information about their own child. **Coordinated and Comprehensive Care for Child and Family** (17 items) assesses whether care is continuous and consistent over time, settings, and people, and whether care is provided for the whole child and family. **Respectful and Supportive Care** (9 items) addresses behaviours that make parents feel they are treated with respect as individuals, equals, and experts. It includes behaviours such as treating each parent as an individual rather than as a "case," and providing enough time to talk so that parents do not feel rushed.

A series of studies have been conducted to ensure that MPOC contains the most appropriate items, and is reliable and valid. Approximately 1,600 parents from 13 children's rehabilitation centres across Ontario participated in the instrument development and validation studies. Details of MPOC's reliability and validity are described in King et al.[14] and a manual has been developed.[15] MPOC displays excellent reliability and validity and has been used in several recent studies.[18-20]

MPOC can be used to measure parent perceptions of important aspects of care on a specific, behavioural level. It is based on interpersonal and informational aspects of care that are important to parents and its five scales reflect what parents view as important service provider behaviours. MPOC's development and content therefore nicely match the current interest in measuring the extent to which services reflect a family-centred approach.

The Family-Centered Program Rating Scale (FamPRS). Service providers' perceptions of the provision of family-centred service were measured using the Family-Centered Program Rating Scale (FamPRS).[21] The FamPRS was developed as a program evaluation tool to assess the family-centred services of early intervention programs. Both a parent version and a service provider version are available. We did not use the parent version of the FamPRS because we had already obtained data on parents' perceptions of caregiving using MPOC (these data were available from the measure's development phase).

The FamPRS scale has 59 statements about features of early intervention programs. These statements capture *how* services are offered as well as *which* services are offered. Respondents are asked to rate on a 4-point scale each feature's importance (from not important to very important) and the performance of their program (from poor to excellent). The FamPRS contains 11 subscales. In our opinion, the labels of these subscales do not completely communicate the content of the subscales. Accordingly, we developed short phrases to capture the fuller meaning of the FamPRS subscales (Table 1). Subscale scores are calculated by averaging responses for the items contained in each subscale.

The factor structure of the FamPRS has been examined, but only for the parent version, and only the factor structure of the importance ratings has been examined, not the ratings of the programs' actual performance. To investigate the dimensions underlying parents' importance ratings, Murphy and Lee[21] conducted a series of principal component analyses. These provided 11 subscales, each measuring a statistically independent aspect of family-centred service. The internal consistency coefficients indicate

TABLE 1. Family-Centered Program Rating Scale (FamPRS): Descriptions of Scales

FamPRS Scale Name	Brief Description* *Items reflect the extent to which programs/services/staff . . .*
Flexibility and Innovation in Programming (6 items)	provide information in a variety of ways to family members
Providing and Coordinating *Responsive* Services (4 items)	assist families in making decisions and obtaining services quickly and easily
Individualizing Services and Ways of Handling Complaints (4 items)	consider the family's practical constraints (around transportation and scheduling) and make them feel comfortable to ask questions and raise concerns
Providing Appropriate and Practical *Information* (11 items)	provide practical information in a way that is not overwhelming and respects differences among families and provides specific information about the child
Communication Timing and Style (4 items)	communicate in a timely, complete, friendly and honest manner
Developing and Maintaining Comfortable *Relationships* (6 items)	develop rapport with family members by asking for feedback, offering home visits, and getting to know them
Building Family-Staff *Collaboration* (5 items)	involve family members in making plans and decisions about services
Respecting the Family as *Decisionmaker* (5 items)	encourage parents to make their own decisions around level of involvement and the services they receive
Respecting the Family's Expertise and *Strengths* (6 items)	treat parents as the experts on their child and consider the strengths of each family
Recognizing the Family's Need for *Autonomy* (5 items)	treat family members with respect (not asking them to repeat information or telling them what they need)
Building Positive *Expectations* (3 items)	provide families with positive views of the future and what they can teach their child

* These descriptions were developed by the authors of the current article, not by the authors of the FamPRS.

that the 11 subscales (based on the parent data) have moderate to high reliability for service providers.

A comparison of the two measurement tools. The MPOC and FamPRS instruments measure somewhat different aspects of family-centred service. We evaluated the match between the scales of the two measures, both on the scale level and on the specific, item-by-item level. Certain scales overlapped well. Both measures have scales that capture the ideas of providing information to parents and encouraging partnership and collaboration with parents (although MPOC has many more partnership items than does the FamPRS). Both measures also tap the ideas of respecting families and providing them with specific information about the child. In some areas, however, no overlap was present. The FamPRS does not emphasize the notion of providing coordinated and comprehensive care; MPOC does not cover the responsiveness of services to families' needs, nor the comfort of the relationship between parents and service providers.

We found very little overlap between the two measures on the item level. Only 18 items had similar content (about 30% of the items in total). In summary, although the overlap between the MPOC and FamPRS on the item level is small and the two measures emphasize different aspects of family-centred service, they do measure conceptually similar aspects of family-centred service.

Samples

Sampling for the parent survey. In 1992, as part of a measure development study for the MPOC, a convenience sample of 1002 parents was recruited from 13 of the 20 children's rehabilitation centres in Ontario. These parents were asked to complete a 101-item questionnaire examining their perceptions of the care they and their children received.

Of the 1002 consenting families, at least one parent from 749 families (74.8%) completed and returned the questionnaire. Due to various exclusions (such as a significant amount of missing or incomplete data, and the inclusion of only one parent per family to maintain the independence of cases), a sample of 653 usable questionnaires was obtained. For the purpose of this article, we then selected only those respondents who indicated that their child received the majority of .their services from one of the rehabilitation centres. This resulted in a total sample of 436 parents.

Sampling for the service provider survey. A convenience sample was obtained by asking clinicians from all 20 rehabilitation centres to participate in a mailed survey conducted in 1994. Letters were sent to the executive directors telling them of the survey and asking them to give survey materials to discipline leaders or program managers. These department heads/managers were asked to give the survey to their staff members, ensuring that at least one senior clinician and one clinician newer to the field were approached.

A total of 572 packages was sent in a single mailing to invite participation from clinicians in 123 departments or programs. The package contained a letter explaining the purpose of the survey, the Family-Centered

Program Rating Scale, a demographic form, and a stamped return envelope. No follow-up reminders could be sent to potential participants. Completed survey forms were received from 309 service providers (a 54% return rate). All 20 centres were represented in the sample, with a range from 3-34 respondents per centre (note that centres ranged in staff size from about 5 to over 150 full-time-equivalent positions).

RESULTS

Parents' Perceptions of Services

Description of parent respondents to MPOC survey. Most of the 436 respondents were mothers (81.9%) and most (84.9%) were from two-parent families. The majority of the mothers (65.1%) and their spouses (58.3%) had education beyond high school and were English-speaking (95.2%). The median total family income was in the range of $45,000 to $59,999 per year (Canadian) which is comparable to the 1990 Ontario population data showing the median husband-wife family income to be $53,217.[22]

The sample included parents of children within a wide age range (7 months to 20 years, with most in the 2 to 12 year age range). The majority (55.6%) were boys. These children represented a wide range of chronic, mostly neurodevelopmental disorders (such as cerebral palsy, developmental delay, and spina bifida). Over half of the children had more than one health or development problem, and over half were receiving multiple therapies (at least two of occupational therapy, physiotherapy, and speech-language therapy).

MPOC survey findings. Table 2 contains the mean scale scores, standard deviations, and number of respondents for the parent sample. A mean score of 4 indicates that on average, parents report that family-centred behaviours "sometimes" occur and a mean score of 7 indicates that the family-centred behaviours occur "to a great extent." The scale scores in Table 2 indicate that parents perceive that centres provide moderately high levels of *Respectful and Supportive Care* (M = 5.85 on the 7-point scale), *Enabling and Partnership* (M = 5.57), and *Coordinated and Comprehensive Care* (M = 5.41).

Relatively speaking, centres do less well at providing information to parents. The mean score of 4.16 on *Providing General Information*, for example, indicates that on average parents report that centre staff "sometimes" meet parents' needs for information. Centres also do less well at *Providing Specific Information about the Child* (M = 5.19).

TABLE 2. Means and Standard Deviations on the MPOC Scales for the Parent Sample

Scales	Number of Items	M	SD	n
Enabling & Partnership	16	5.57	1.07	424
Providing General Information	9	4.16	1.56	385
Providing Specific Information about the Child	5	5.19	1.41	394
Coordinated & Comprehensive Care for Child and Family	17	5.41	1.24	404
Respectful & Supportive Care	9	5.85	1.07	430

More detailed information about service delivery is provided by the individual items on each scale. Table 3 presents items on which at least one third of the 436 parents indicated that the behaviour occurred "sometimes" or less. For each of these 14 items, the table contains the percent of parents who indicated that a behaviour occurred "never" to "sometimes" (points 1 to 4) and the percent who indicated it occurred more than "sometimes" (points 5 to 7). We believed that behaviours occurring "sometimes" or less for one third of the parents (a substantial proportion) were problematic behaviours that managers and service providers would be interested in considering. They could use this information to identify areas in which services could be improved.

Of the 14 items occurring "sometimes" or less, 9 (64%) are from the *Providing General Information* scale. These items deal with a wide range of information needs: information about disability, how to contact other parents, information on the types of services available at the centre and in the community, and advice on how to get information. Two other items deal with *Providing Specific Information about the Child*. The majority of the "problem" items, therefore, deal with information provision.

Service Providers' Perceptions of Services

Description of service provider respondents to FamPRS survey. The service provider sample included clinicians from a wide variety of disciplines. The majority were from speech-language pathology (21%), physiotherapy (19%), occupational therapy (19%), early childhood education (10%), and social work (8%). Half of the respondents had been in pediatric practice less than 10 years while 38% had practiced for 10 or more years

TABLE 3. MPOC Items on Which at Least One-Third of Parents Indicated the Behaviour Occurred "Sometimes" or Less

Item **To what extent do the people who work with your child . . .**	Scale Name	% Responding "Sometimes" or Less*	% Responding More than "Sometimes"**
have information available about your child's disability (e.g., its causes, how it progresses, future outlook)?	Providing General Information	53.4	36.3
promote family-to-family gatherings for social, informational or shared experiences?	Providing General Information	51.9	33.4
have information available to you in various forms, such as a booklet, kit, video, etc.?	Providing General Information	50.7	40.9
provide opportunities for the entire family to obtain information?	Providing General Information	48.4	30.9
make you feel like a partner in your child's care?	Enabling & Partnership	47.0	49.6
give you information about the types of services offered at the Centre or in your community?	Providing General Information	46.9	45.6
provide opportunities for special guests to speak to parents on topics of interest?	Providing General Information	45.6	36.8
make themselves available to you as a resource (e.g., emotional support, advocacy, information)?	Coordinated & Comprehensive Care	43.8	44.9
provide support to help cope with the impact of childhood disability (e.g., by advocating on your behalf or informing you of assistance programs)?	Providing General Information	43.3	38.6
provide advice on how to get information or to contact other parents (e.g., Centre's parent resource library)?	Providing General Information	42.7	50.7
tell you about the results from assessments?	Providing Specific Information about the Child	40.9	48.1

TABLE 3 (continued)

Item **To what extent do the people who work with your child . . .**	Scale Name	% Responding "Sometimes" or Less*	% Responding More than "Sometimes"**
have general information available about different concerns (e.g., financial costs or assistance, genetic counselling, dating and sexuality)?	Providing General Information	40.6	40.4
offer you positive feedback or encouragement (e.g., in carrying out a home program)?	Enabling & Partnership	38.7	54.8
explain what they are doing when you are watching your child in therapy?	Providing Specific Information about the Child	37.4	60.2

* values of 1-4 on the 7-point scale
** values of 5-7 on the 7-point scale
Note. Percentages may not add to 100% due to items being answered as "not applicable" or omitted.

(12% did not respond to this question). Thirty-two percent worked pre-dominantly with infants and preschool age children, 29% with predomi-nantly pre-adolescents and adolescents, and 36% worked with all age groups. Most (74%) indicated that they are employed full-time.

FamPRS survey findings. Data from the FamPRS survey were inter-preted in several ways. Graphic profiles of the mean importance and performance data for the 11 subscales were examined for all rehabilitation centres combined. A visual analysis was completed to inspect each graph-ic profile for similarities and differences. Visual inspection of data profiles also was completed for results coded by years of pediatric practice and part-time versus fulltime work status to determine the influences of these factors on family-centred service. We did not perform statistical compari-sons due to the exploratory nature of the surveys and the fact we did not have specific hypotheses to test.

Following visual analysis, we examined differences between impor-tance scores and perceived performance scores. Specifically, we identified subscales in which mean perceived performance was scored 0.60 or more below the mean importance rating for that subscale (0.60 was chosen because it represented the average variability or standard deviation of the mean score for all subscales).

The FamPRS profile across the 20 Ontario rehabilitation centres is displayed in Figures 1 and 2. From the data in the two figures, service providers clearly considered all subscales of the FamPRS to be important for their programs. Highest value was placed on Providing and Coordinating *Responsive* Services, *Communication* Timing and Style, Respecting the Family's Expertise and *Strengths*, and Building Positive *Expectations*. Service providers reported that their performance for most subscales ranged from "okay" (a score of 2) to "good" (a score of 3). Performance was perceived to be better on subscales that were rated as more important. Three subscales (*Communication* Timing and Style, Respecting the Family's Expertise and *Strengths*, and Building Positive *Expectations*) received scores of "good." The lowest performance score was found on *Flexibility* and Innovation in Programming (which received a score of "okay").

On four subscales the difference between the importance and the performance scores was above 0.60: *Flexibility* and Innovation in Programming, Building Family-Staff *Collaboration*, Providing and Coordinating *Responsive* Services, and *Individualizing* Services and Ways of Handling Complaints.

FamPRS profiles also were examined by years of practice, years of practice with children, part-time or full-time work status of respondents, and work at a small or larger rehabilitation centre. Small centres were

FIGURE 1. Average Importance and Performance Scores for the First Six FamPRS Scales

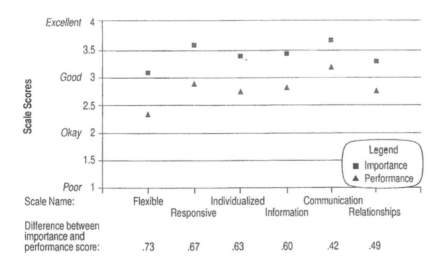

FIGURE 2. Average Importance and Performance Scores for the Remaining Five FamPRS Scales

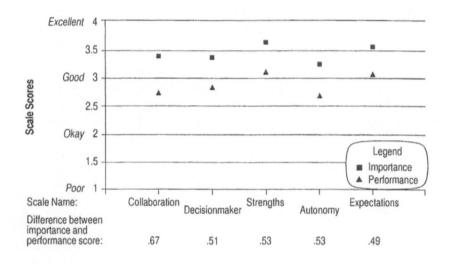

defined as those that had fewer than 30 full-time-equivalent staff positions. Visual examination of the importance and performance data indicated that none of these factors made a difference in the data profiles. For example, the data profiles for smaller centres were virtually identical to the profiles for larger centres.

DISCUSSION

A Comparison of Parents' and Service Providers' Perceptions

Comparisons between parents' and service providers' perceptions of the level of family-centred service are scarce[12] but potentially very useful. Difficulties can arise if parents and service providers have appreciably different perceptions of the level of family-centred service. For example, service providers may believe they are providing a good level of family-centred service, but parents may be dissatisfied. Parents may feel little control over the decisions that are made about their child's treatment or may feel they are not treated with respect or consideration for their family's circumstances.

The two surveys we conducted provide a "snapshot" view of the family-centredness of care and services in Ontario children's rehabilitation centres. Of interest is that both parents and service providers identify the same areas of relative strength and weakness. Both groups reported that the interpersonal aspects of service delivery were done well. On the Measure of Processes of Care, parents gave the highest ratings to *Enabling and Partnership* and to *Respectful and Supportive Care*. On the Family-Centered Program Rating Scale, service providers indicated that they were doing well at communicating with parents in a timely, complete, friendly and honest manner (*Communication* Timing and Style), treating parents as the experts on their child and considering the strengths of each family (Respecting the Family's Expertise and *Strengths*), and providing families with positive views of the future and what they can teach their child (Building Positive *Expectations*). The staffs of children's rehabilitation centres in Ontario, therefore, appear to be doing a good job in meeting parents' needs to be involved in decision-making about their child's services, to be treated respectfully and supportively, dealt with in a friendly and honest manner, and provided with a positive view of the future. Parents report fairly high levels of the occurrence of caregiving behaviours that reflect how they are treated in interpersonal interactions with service providers, and service providers themselves report that they are doing a good job interpersonally.

Both groups indicated that the provision of information was a relatively weak area. On the MPOC, parents gave the lowest ratings to *Providing General Information* and *Providing Specific Information about the Child*. On the FamPRS, service providers indicated they were doing least well at providing information in a variety of ways to family members (*Flexibility* and Innovation in Programming). Improvements, therefore, could be made in the area of information provision. This could include providing information about available services (in the centre and the community), the nature of disabilities, how to contact other families of children with similar needs, and other issues of importance to families.

Several limitations of our survey study need to be mentioned. We compared parents' and service providers' perceptions using two different measures and the two surveys were conducted approximately two years apart. Any differences in the perceptions of parents and service providers could be due to these measurement and time differences; however, as discussed above, the surveys revealed strong similarities in the perceptions of service providers and parents. These findings parallel those of von Essen and Sjödén[12] who found that patients and staff members made similar rankings of the occurrence of caring behaviours.

Discrepancies Between Importance and Performance Scores on the FamPRS

We found relatively large discrepancies between service providers' perceptions of the importance and performance scores on four subscales of the FamPRS. According to von Essen and Sjödén,[12] staff perceptions of important caring behaviours may not be accurate predictors of what staff actually do. They did not find significant associations between staff's perceptions of the occurrence and importance of caring behaviours.

Why do these discrepancies exist? Most likely, service providers are unable to provide care in the ways they would like. In the present study, the biggest discrepancies between judged importance and self-reported occurrence involved: providing information in a variety of ways to families (*Flexibility* and Innovation in Programming), involving family members in making plans and decisions about services (Building Family-Staff *Collaboration*), assisting families in making decisions and obtaining services quickly and easily (Providing and Coordinating *Responsive* Services), and considering the family's practical constraints and making them feel comfortable to ask questions and raise concerns (*Individualizing* Services and Ways of Handling Complaints). These four aspects of family-centred service may be the most difficult for service providers to implement because they involve close collaboration with others (including the family), or networking with other service agencies, and may be seen by management as less efficient ways of providing services.

Implications

The findings of this study are consistent with some new directions in service delivery that are currently taking place within Ontario children's rehabilitation centres. The findings indicate that service providers believe that it is important to provide family-centred services and confirm that centres are doing well in various aspects of this. It is obvious that these centres need to focus on information provision. One way that many centres are meeting this need is by setting up resource centres to help meet parents' needs for information. Other methods could include encouraging development of parent support groups and parent networking, and providing information nights and written resource materials.

The similarities between service providers' and parents' perceptions should not be taken to mean that we can ask only service providers (or parents) for their perceptions; the perspectives of both parties must be assessed. The similarities we have noted are on the larger level (i.e., good interpersonal treatment but relatively weak information provision), and differences might be found if comparisons were made on the level of individual behaviours.

For individual centres, data from service providers and parents could provide important information about how well a centre is achieving its vision or meeting its goals. For example, a centre may value service responsiveness much more than providing practical information. One, therefore, would expect parents (and service providers) to indicate that they received (or provided) responsive services to a much higher extent than practical information. If this were not the case, then efforts should be directed at bringing the reality in line with the centre's values.

Centre staff members clearly report a considerable degree of support for the ideas of family-centred service; however, in some areas, big discrepancies exist between what service providers see as important and what they actually do. This may reflect the difficulty in implementing some of the aspects of family-centred service that deal with service coordination, joint decision-making, and service responsiveness. Additional effort may be needed to address the most challenging aspects of professional-client relationships if we are to continue on the road toward "family-centredness." Speculating about methods to foster the implementation of family-centred service is interesting. Among other things, these methods will undoubtedly include training service providers to become familiar with the concepts of family-centred service and proficient in problem-solving, conflict resolution, and negotiation.

Utility of the Measurement Tools

We believe that MPOC is a useful tool for centres interested in knowing the extent to which parents view services as family-centred and wishing to identify those aspects of service that could be improved. MPOC could be used in program evaluation studies and total quality management activities, directed either at a centre as a whole or at a specific program, or at specific services offered within a program. MPOC provides useful scale and item information about the frequency of occurrence of family-centred behaviours that are important to parents.

The FamPRS measure provides useful information about service providers' perceptions of family-centred services and about discrepancies between the importance and occurrence of specific family-centred behaviours; however, it has several limitations. It was designed for early intervention programs, although its items seem to apply to all age ranges. More reliability and validity evidence is needed; this scale is relatively new (published in 1991). As well, the names provided for the subscales do not always represent their content accurately, and so the subscale data are difficult to interpret. The utility of the FamPRS in children's rehabilitation centres has been examined only once previously in a study at the Hugh MacMillan Rehabilitation Centre in Ontario.[23] The investigators found that the scale provided a good basis for discussion of training needs and program goals in family-centred services but was not useful to evaluate change in family-centred service over time.

Future Research Directions

A number of factors (e.g., centre size, years of practice of service providers) did not influence the way in which service providers responded to the FamPRS. For instance, service providers' style of interacting with family members did not appear to be related to the number of years of experience he or she had providing rehabilitation services to children. And larger centres did not provide more "family-centred" services than did smaller ones (or vice versa). These findings may indicate that perceptions of the family-centredness of service are influenced more by the climate or culture of a centre than by the training or experience of service providers or structural aspects of centres. Future research to examine the influence of centre leadership and culture on the adoption of family-centred practices may be useful.

The surveys have provided baseline information on perceptions of the "family-centredness" of service delivery in children's rehabilitation centres in Ontario. These observations will be useful if the surveys are readministered again at a later date. Many Ontario children's rehabilitation centres are adopting a more family-centred approach to service provision. Readministration of the surveys would allow us to see whether changes in service delivery actually do change parents' and staff members' perceptions of services and programs. Because neither the FamPRS nor MPOC was developed as an evaluative measure, we do not currently know whether these measures are capable of reflecting true change over time. This is an issue for further exploration as we continue to examine the family-centredness of rehabilitation services provided to children in Ontario.

The generalizability and relevance of this survey study's findings to children's rehabilitation centres outside of Ontario is unknown. We do not know whether the pattern of good interpersonal treatment but relatively weak information provision is one that would characterize rehabilitation services in other locations. In this article, however, we provide a useful example of how to measure the level of family-centred service in children's rehabilitation centres (and provide information on the utility of two possible measurement tools) and discuss the practical utility of such an endeavour.

REFERENCES

1. Dunst CJ, Trivette CM, Deal AG. *Supporting and Strengthening Families (Vol. 1): Methods, Strategies and Practices.* Cambridge, MA: Brookline Books; 1994.

2. Rogers CR. *Client-centered Therapy.* Cambridge, MA: Brookline Books; 1951.

3. Abramson JS. Enhancing patient participation: clinical strategies in the discharge planning process. *Soc Work Health Care.* 1990;14:53-71.

4. Rosenbaum P, King S, Law M, King G, Evans J. Family-centred service: A conceptual framework and research review. *Phys Occup Ther Pediatr.* 1988; 18(1):1-20.

5. Dunst CJ, Trivette CM, Davis M, Cornwall J. Enabling and empowering families of children with health impairments. *Child Health Care.* 1988;17:71-81.

6. Bazyk S. Changes in attitudes and beliefs regarding parent participation and home programs: An update. *Am J Occup Ther.* 1989;43:723-728.

7. Law M. The environment: A focus for occupational therapy. *Can J Occup Ther.* 1991;58:171-179.

8. Moxley-Haegert L, Serbin LA. Developmental education for parents of delayed infants: Effects on parental motivation and children's development. *Child Dev.* 1983;54:1324-1331.

9. Stein REK, Jessop DJ. Does pediatric home care make a difference for children with chronic illness? Findings from the pediatric ambulatory care treatment study. *Pediatrics.* 1984; 73:845-853.

10. Stein REK, Jessop DJ. Long-term mental health effects of a pediatric home care program. *Pediatrics.* 1991;88:490-496.

11. Cleary PD, Edgman-Levitan S, Roberts M, Moloney TW, McMullen W, Walker JD, Delbanco TL. Patients evaluate their hospital care: a national survey. *Health Aff.* 1991;Winter: 254-267.

12. von Essen L, Sjödén P. Perceived occurrence and importance of caring behaviours among patients and staff in psychiatric, medical and surgical care. *J Adv Nurs.* 1995;21:266-276.

13. Mahoney G, O'Sullivan P, Dennebaum J. Maternal perceptions of early intervention services: a scale for assessing family-focused intervention. *Top Early Child Spec Educ.* 1990;10:1-15.

14. King S, Rosenbaum P, King G. Parents' perceptions of care-giving: development and validation of a measure of processes. *Dev Med Child Neurol.* 1996; 38:757-772.

15. King S, Rosenbaum P, King G. *The Measure of Processes of Care: A Means to Assess Family-centred Behaviours of Health Care Providers.* Unpublished manual. Hamilton, Ontario: McMaster University, Neurodevelopmental Clinical Research Unit; 1995.

16. Rosenbaum P, King S, Cadman D. Measuring processes of caregiving to physically disabled children and their families: I: Identifying relevant components of care. *Dev Med Child Neurol.* 1992;34:103-114.

17. Baine S, Rosenbaum P, King S. Chronic childhood illnesses: what aspects of caregiving do parents value? *Child Care Health Dev.* 1995;21:291-304.

18. King G, King S, Rosenbaum P. How mothers and fathers view professional caregiving for children with disabilities. *Dev Med Child Neurol.* 1996;38:397-407.

19. King G, Rosenbaum P, King S. Evaluating family-centred service using a measure of parents' perceptions. *Child Care Health Dev.* In press.

20. Rosenbaum P, King S, King G. *Parental values about caregiving: Is there a relationship with sociodemographic factors?* Manuscript in preparation; 1996.

21. Murphy DL, Lee IM. *Family-Centered Program Rating Scale: User's Manual,* ed 2. Lawrence, KS: Beach Center on Families and Disability, The University of Kansas; 1991.

22. Statistics Canada. *Selected income statistics* (1991 Census of Canada, Catalogue number 93-331). Ottawa, ON: Industry, Science and Technology Canada; 1993.

23. Gan C, Greenberg J, Lord J, Jutai J. *Family-centred service development project.* Toronto, ON: Hugh MacMillan Rehabilitation Centre, unpublished; 1994.

The Family-Centred Approach
to Providing Services:
A Parent Perspective

Linda Viscardis

SUMMARY. In this paper information is brought together from literature about family-centred service and the perceptions and feelings of parents who want a system that is responsive to their family's needs. It is written by a parent who advocates for parents as equal partners in the provision of services to families and their children who have disabilities. Parents whose children need specialized services believe that they are best able to make decisions regarding services they receive. With the support of the service provider, parents will be able to identify their roles as members on their child's team. With continued support, parents will fulfill this role, learn new skills and become empowered to take control over the service plan. Parents will become positive role models for children who may then learn the value of becoming active partners of their teams. *[Article copies available for a fee from The Haworth Document Delivery Service: 1-800-342-9678. E-mail address: getinfo@haworthpressinc.com]*

Linda Viscardis, BA, is Team Leader and Community Development Worker, Peterborough Family Enrichment Centre. She is Co-Founder of P.R.O.S.P.E.C.T.S., a support and advocacy group for families who have children with special needs.

Address correspondence to: Linda Viscardis, BA, 664 Pinewood Drive, Peterborough, ON, Canada K9K 1L2.

The author would like to acknowledge the following parents who provided input for this paper: Christine Cannon, Karen Galloro, Rosemary Smith, and Suzette White.

[Haworth co-indexing entry note]: "The Family-Centred Approach to Providing Services: A Parent Perspective." Viscardis, Linda. Co-published simultaneously in *Physical & Occupational Therapy in Pediatrics* (The Haworth Press, Inc.) Vol. 18, No. 1, 1998, pp. 41-53; and: *Family-Centred Assessment and Intervention in Pediatric Rehabilitation* (ed: Mary Law) The Haworth Press, Inc., 1998, pp. 41-53. Single or multiple copies of this article are available for a fee from The Haworth Document Delivery Service [1-800-342-9678, 9:00 a.m. - 5:00 p.m. (EST). E-mail address: getinfo@haworthpressinc.com].

In the past several years, the term "family-centred" has been tossed around like a hot potato. It is a relatively new concept that, at times, appears, like the potato, too hot to handle. The concept presents service providers with the challenge of finding new ways of doing business, while presenting families with the opportunity to have more involvement in how services are provided to their family. This paper is written from a parent's perspective with the belief that the very foundation of a family-centred approach to the provision of services is that families have the strength, capacity, ability, right and responsibility to learn about their options and make informed choices and decisions as partners with the people who work with them and their children. The fact that this paper was requested is an indication of the increased acknowledgment that families have a lot to say about how their needs should be met.

In this paper I will describe the parent perspective as it relates to aspects of family-centred service that have been defined in the literature: where the concept came from; what a family-centred approach is; what the key elements of family-centred service are; what the barriers to a family-centred approach are; what needs to change; what some strategies for implementing a family-centred approach are, and what outcomes can be anticipated with a family-centred approach. Parents' and service providers' perspectives quoted in the paper were obtained from questionnaires completed by several service providers, as well as parents whose children have been labelled "disabled." The questionnaire was based on The University of Kansas, Beach Center on Families and Disability's Family-Centered Program Rating Scale[1] and was administered by the author.

ORIGINS OF THE FAMILY-CENTRED SERVICE CONCEPT

In the past, the service provider was considered the expert. Families deferred decisions to the professionals who set goals which focused on making changes in the child. During the past decade, awareness of the role of the family in the child's life has increased. The family is now recognized as the constant in the child's life while professionals will come and go. Because families are the constant in their child's life, parents know their child best and have much insight to offer into what and how services should be provided. Parent advocates continue to stress the importance of services being provided in a way that meets the needs of the whole family. By providing services that suit the whole family, a greater probability exists that the needs of the child will be met. As more parents speak up about their expectations about being involved in the care of their child, required changes in the system are being identified, discussed, and implemented. Nevertheless, much work remains to be done in various human service sectors, as the following quotes from families make clear.

> As our son grows, many people will come and go, however, our family will remain the same. Decisions we make for our child must reflect goals we have for him, otherwise our values will be compromised. To our family, service providers are our greatest resource who, after having given us all pertinent information, must respect our ability to make decisions that will enhance our child's strengths.

Parents, eager to become more involved in their child's team, become frustrated with the pace of change in some service sectors.

> I can't understand why my support worker sees so clearly what my family needs when my daughter's (other service provider) cannot. I want all of my daughter's team members to be at the same level of understanding. I know that if only all team members understood my family like my support worker understands them my life would be so much easier. I feel like the burden for making things change is on my shoulders. I want to be the leader of my daughter's team but sometimes I just get so frustrated with the system's inability to adapt quickly to my family's needs. I don't have time for this–I already have enough to worry about.

It is informed, involved and questioning parents who will propel this movement forward. A danger must be avoided as the system evolves. In their eagerness, agencies adapt their working styles, their programs and services to respond to the need for more parent involvement. As more parents become involved with support groups, as support groups become involved with agencies, and as agencies work toward including parents in decision-making, families are often expected to take on a new and more complex role. Confusion arises when, as the movement toward family-centredness gains momentum, service providers see parents who are unwilling or unable to take on the role of a key player in their child's team. Service providers confuse "family driven" with "family centred," and become frustrated when all parents do not fit their agency's definition of "team member." Often, in a newly evolving family-centred environment, parents may be expected to become the team leader, or at the very least, the constant who pulls all the services together. Service providers may have difficulty accepting that not all parents are willing or able to assume these responsibilities. Agencies must not, in the name of family-centred service, dump responsibilities on parents without being sensitive to the parents' willingness or ability to be involved. Service providers must be aware of where the family is in the adaptation and diagnosis process and provide support for, not control over, the family's involvement.

A truly family-centred approach is one where families are given options about the intensity of their involvement as a team member. The service should be designed to meet the needs of the whole family, and if that means that the team leader is a paid agency/support person, then that is what should be provided. Parents must be encouraged to define their role in their child's team for themselves. This role must be allowed to be fulfilled in an environment of acceptance, non-judgment and support. The role of service providers then, is to ensure that this environment is sustained.

WHAT IS A FAMILY-CENTRED APPROACH– HOW IS IT DEFINED?

A group of parents in Peterborough, Ontario (members of P.R.O.S.P.E.C.T.S., a support and advocacy group for families who have children with special needs) got together a few years ago with staff from the local children's rehabilitation centre to talk about how the term "family-centred approach" might be defined. After much discussion, these people agreed that the family-centred approach is one that "*begins with the child's and family's strengths, needs and hopes, and results in a service plan which responds to the needs of the whole family. It involves education, support, direct services and self-help approaches. The role of the service provider is to support, encourage and enhance the competence of parents in their role as caregivers.*" Parents believe that services that are planned, defined and provided to meet an *agency's* needs, or even only the *child's* needs, without consideration of the entire *family's* needs, will inconsistently meet the family's expectations. If an agency's needs are met while the family's are not, then the services are at risk of being inflexible and inappropriate. In such an environment, the family *may* feel that their needs are adequately being met, but more likely they will feel let down, overwhelmed, frustrated, or even angry. Because the service is designed to meet the agency's needs, suggestions for improvement or even complaints will have little chance of having any effect. Parents in this situation will often appear disinterested, unmotivated, non-compliant or hysterical. Parents, whose needs are not being met and who are not dealing well with the situation, are quickly labelled by service providers as "difficult." This labelling often undermines the parent's authority as leader of their child's team.

Dunst, Johanson, Trivette and Hamby state that the term "family-centred" refers to "a combination of beliefs and practices that define particular ways of working with families that are consumer-driven and competency enhancing,"[2(p 115)] and that in a family-centred approach "families' needs and desires determine all aspects of service delivery and resource provision. Professionals are seen as the agents and instruments of families, and intervene in ways that maximally promote family decision making, capabilities, and competencies."[2(p 118)]

At a presentation about delivering services for children with special needs and their families, Nancy Draper reported that the Kennedy Institute on the Family defines a family-centred approach to service delivery as a "collaborative relationship between families and professionals in the continual pursuit of being responsive to the priorities and choices of families."[3] The challenge is for service providers and families to see how their specific situation fits into this definition and to move forward using this definition as a guideline for decision-making.

Despite the existence of various definitions, the term "family-centred" does not necessarily mean that all sectors know how to relate the concept to their way of doing business. The term means different things at various times to different people and different sectors. A service provider's perspective of what makes a service family-centred may differ considerably from that of the family receiving the service. For example, when asked to rate how well surprises are avoided when dealing with information about children, a service provider indicated that in this program surprises are avoided by parents having "regular communication with the (service provider)"–the program was rated "good" at doing this. The parent perspective on this same question was that surprises are avoided "only when parents ask repeatedly for this to happen"–the program was rated "poor" at doing this. Apparently, the definition of "family-centred service" is not the same for the two individuals rating this identical service.

> Imagine my horror when, after six years of involvement with this service provider, I suddenly heard a new label being placed on my daughter. I simply was not prepared for this and found myself struggling for composure instead of participating in the case conference. When confronted about this, the service provider was very nonchalant. He did not acknowledge my concern at all. I don't think he even realized why I was so upset!

Parents believe that the foundation of a family-centred approach to the provision of services is that families are capable of making informed choices and decisions as partners with the people who work with them and their children, and that as the primary care provider parents have the right and the responsibility to do so. A family-centred approach is one that accommodates this belief by providing a forum for truly interactive communication between parties in a respectful and growth-oriented environment.

WHAT ARE THE KEY ELEMENTS
OF FAMILY-CENTRED SERVICE?

The National Centre for Family-Centred Care,[4] identifies the following key elements of family-centred care in a pamphlet published by The Association for the Care of Children's Health:

- "recognizing that the family is the constant in a child's life, while the service systems and personnel within those systems fluctuate;
- "facilitating parent/professional collaboration at all levels of health care: care of an individual child; program development, implementation, and evaluation; and policy formation;
- "honouring the racial, ethnic, cultural, and socioeconomic diversity of families;
- "recognizing family strengths and individuality and respecting different methods of coping;
- "sharing with parents complete and unbiased information on a continuing basis and in a supportive manner;
- "encouraging and facilitating family-to-family support and networking;
- "understanding and incorporating the developmental needs of infants, children, adolescents, and their families into health care systems;
- "implementing comprehensive policies and programs that provide emotional and financial support to meet the needs of families;
- "designing accessible health care systems that are flexible, culturally competent, and responsive to family-identified needs."

Parents feel that in a family-centred environment, service providers and parents are in tune with one another's positions. If this happens, there is little to no disparity in providers' perceptions of what is important to families. As one parent indicated in the questionnaire, "*This System needs desperately to improve communication between (agency) and family.*" Although the service provider noted that "regular home-(agency) communication is essential," he or she also indicated that the agency has a "problem of availability of time." Families believe that, in a family-centred environment, the "problem of availability of time" would be satisfactorily dealt with in order to be responsive to the family's needs. In a family-centred environment, if the problem is not resolved, then there is a comfortable way to work out disagreements between families and service providers. Using this same pair of individuals as an example, it is obvious that differing perspectives get in the way of the service being family-centred. This service provider believes that the service is "good" at providing a "comfortable way to work out disagreements," whereas the parent rates this activity as "poor." Because of the difference in perspectives, little chance exists that the service will improve without the parents becoming assertive in an effort to be heard and understood.

> I believe that parents and service providers all have to realize that to disagree does not mean to be disagreeable. We all have to be open to ideas and suggestions and the possibility that despite past experience or training, no one person has all the answers, and that's OK.

Parents do not necessarily describe an agency or a service as "family-centred," but are very quick to identify an agency or service that meets their needs well. When asked "What are ways in which this program or service could be more helpful and welcoming to families; what are some of the barriers to a family-centred approach?" parents who rated a program or service highly indicated that there were very few ways that improvements could be made:

> I can honestly say that I have not encountered any barriers. The (program) takes my concerns and suggestions very seriously and every effort is made to address or carry them out.

Parents who rated a program or service poorly had various suggestions for improvement:

> I want to be considered an equal partner of my child's team. I want to feel welcome. I want the service providers to seek my help, advice and ideas. I want them to respond to my concerns quickly. I want communication to be prompt, friendly and helpful. I want to feel that I can approach them with any concern and be heard.

> I don't want to have to tell my story over and over again. I want the system to be coordinated so that all the people who need to know my story already know it.

I want the service providers to understand that with their help I can decide what my family needs. I don't want to have to beg, cajole, or manipulate to get what I need. I want services to be easily and readily available. I want the service provider to be able to understand my situation and to be able to give me information about all options open to me. I want the service provider to support me in developing and implementing a plan that meets the needs of my whole family.

Parents want to be taken seriously and given credit for the valuable part they play on their child's team.

The idea that a knowledgeable parent is unable to contribute to solutions is unfounded. . . . For the most part we need (the service provider's) expertise, however, their expertise must be flexible to fit with my child's changing needs.

Families know that a program or service provider that uses a family-centred approach truly makes a difference in the family's ability to cope with day-to-day stresses.

I have to say that all the therapy has helped my daughter to come a long way, but I really think the support we got as a family was even more important. By supporting what I was trying to do with my daughter, our therapist helped me to believe in myself. The staff responded to the needs of my whole family, not just my daughter's. When I was at my wit's end, I took my daughter in for therapy and spent the whole time unloading on our therapist instead. She just listened. And that's just what I needed.

WHAT ARE SOME BARRIERS
TO A FAMILY-CENTRED APPROACH?

Friesen and Koroloff identify four barriers to a family-centred system: "efforts have tended to focus primarily on the child as the unit of services, rather than on the family; efforts have tended to focus primarily on (specific) health services, rather than considering the full range of services needed by the child and family; efforts have tended to emphasize formal services, often ignoring the support provided by informal networks; and the resources and expertise of parents and other family members have not been used."[5(p 13)] Agencies and institutions know that a family-centred approach is the trend, but they may have no clear definition or guidelines specific to their own service, no mandate to change, and therefore they struggle with how to proceed. What seems to be missing in some agencies is a strong commitment to family-centred service on the part of the policy makers. Parents know that they want a louder voice and should be more involved with how a service is defined, but they, too, are often uncertain about how to proceed. They may approach service providers and state their expectations, but service providers will often struggle with how to be flexible in meeting families' needs while meeting their own administrative and policy demands.

Families tend to approach issues related to service delivery in a very straightforward way. They know what they want because they know what will work for them and for their child. They tend to focus on what works for them, rather than the barriers that prevent them from being satisfied with a service. Families who identify a high degree of satisfaction with the services received indicate that:

- the service providers respect differences among children, families and families' ways of life; service providers acknowledge that they don't know what it is like to be in the family's situation;
- parents are acknowledged as the constant in the child's life and as such are recognized as knowing their child best;
- parents are considered equal members of the child's team when the service is being developed, reviewed or changed;
- families' choices and decisions are respected;
- services are planned with families' scheduling needs in mind; service providers acknowledge that they may provide only a portion of the service to a family and that in many cases there are other priorities in the family's life;
- service providers have found a way to balance the family's need for information with the need for support; informal supports are offered (e.g., information about peer support);
- services can change quickly when families' or children's needs change.

All of these things require that an agency, program, service and staff be flexible in order to meet the needs of families. Programs and services must be consumer-driven, but to change a system quickly is difficult. Large bureaucracies such as school boards or hospitals have difficulty in being flexible in adapting to the evolving needs of families. Service providers are often limited in their ability to provide a family-centred service by government mandates and collective agreements between their agency's management and union. Consumer-driven initiatives may be devalued or considered unreasonable in light of the inflexibility of the agency. In an agency-driven model of service, families and children must fit into the program, rather than the program or service fitting the needs of the family and child. Changes in program priorities or staffing happen to meet agency agenda in spite of the needs of the family, resulting in a service which may frustrate parents and not meet the needs of the child.

> The system poses a constant, up hill struggle for me as a parent. The service is often inconsistent, uncoordinated and not always dependable. The frequent change in service providers fragments the service and finds me always having to repeat my daughter's needs which I find exhausting.

A family-centred service is one that removes barriers to families being decision-making partners. It is one that acknowledges that parents are not *just* parents, but rather that parents have strengths, capacities and abilities that must be considered resources by the service provider. A family-centred approach focuses on assets and capabilities, and supports families in strengthening their ability to be contributing members of the team.

> I knew what my daughter needed–I just didn't know how to get it. I knew that, of all the people on the team, I know my child best. I believe I have a right to expect that I will have a say about what services will be provided and that those services will meet my child's and my family's needs. I have realized that the biggest barrier to my involvement in decision-making has been an attitude that parents are not capable of being equal partners. The challenge is to find a way to get past this barrier so that we are all considered full partners in providing a service that meets everyone's needs.

WHAT NEEDS TO CHANGE?

Parents believe that agencies with policies, procedures and services that are driven by service users will have fewer barriers that interfere with implementing a family-centred approach than agencies that do not recognize and work with families as partners. This requires a fundamental shift from the belief that service is provided by professionals to a family because the family is unable to solve the problem themselves, to the belief that service is provided by professionals because the family has identified a need and a service that can meet that need. The professional's role then becomes the provider of a service that exists only to meet the needs identified by families. The service becomes consumer-driven as opposed to agency- or professional-driven. Until service providers accept parents as full partners, a family-centred approach to the delivery of services is unlikely to be successful.

STRATEGIES FOR IMPLEMENTING
A FAMILY-CENTRED APPROACH

Birkmeier[6] suggests the following strategies for implementing a family-centred approach to services for families who have children with special needs:

- service providers should acknowledge the grieving and adaptation process: be able to explain the process, be compassionate, warm and understanding;
- professionals should let parents describe what they want their child to be able to do, to identify goals;
- professionals should focus on the positive aspects of the child;
- service providers should put the parents first and then their child; remember that in order to help them to deal effectively and cope with caring for the child, the parents must feel that they are cared for also;
- professionals should tell parents frequently that they are doing a good job;
- parents should be given an opportunity to meet other parents in similar circumstances;
- professionals should be sensitive and show understanding of the normal adaptation process in response to the loss of a dream for a perfect child; this will enhance their ability to affect positive changes in the child and in the parents' ability to care for the child.

Parents believe, again, that families have the strength, capacity, ability, right and responsibility to learn about their options and make informed choices and decisions as partners with the people who work with them and their children. If service providers also believe this, then a family-centred approach to service will naturally emerge.

WHAT ARE THE OUTCOMES
OF A FAMILY-CENTRED APPROACH?

In an environment of shrinking financial resources, providing only services that best meet the needs of consumers is sensible. We can no longer afford the luxury of providing services just for the sake of providing employment or statistics for bureaucrats. In a family-centred environment, in order to determine the needs, consumers will be an information resource, members of the service provision team. Ideally, this will happen at several levels: consumers, families, or parents will be represented at the level of governance so that decisions will be made that truly accommodate the needs of families; when hiring staff, agencies will make every effort to recruit individuals who can bring a family perspective to the agency's service provision; when recruiting volunteers, every effort will be made to access people who receive, or have received in the past, the services offered by the agency; when providing services to families, parents will be supported in identifying their role as a team member and then in fulfilling that role.

To make this happen, will require a change in attitude–consumers, families, or parents will be treated as equal members of the team; tokenism and condescension will be obliterated. Parents will be supported in acquiring and maintaining skills that will benefit both their families and the agencies whose services they use. Services will be easily and readily accessible and families will know how and when to access them. The needs of families will be put ahead of the needs of service providers. As the needs of families are identified, understood and validated, parents will become more confident in their role as both caregivers and team members. With an increase in confidence and involvement, parents, and agencies, will become better equipped to meet the needs of families in the future. When needs are met consistently, in a supportive, nurturing and family-centred way, families with special needs will be better able to live their lives as normally as other families whose needs are not labelled "special."

When the service system becomes truly family-centred, service providers and agencies will consistently acknowledge that the parent's involvement in decision-making is a life-long responsibility–that parents cannot quit or go on vacation or move on to another "career." They will acknowledge that families do have the capacity to learn about all options available to them and then to make informed choices and decisions as partners with the people who work with them and their children. Service providers and agencies will acknowledge that they are providing a service to meet a need identified by families and that they are in the field to serve families. They will continue to evolve in the family-centredness of their approach to provision of services.

Families ultimately want to take control of their situations so they can better provide for their children. A key outcome of family-centred service is that parents become more skilled and empowered to take control. They learn the skill of advocacy. They become positive role models for their children–many of whom will observe and learn to advocate for themselves when they become adults. These adult "children" will become more able to take control over their lives. They will become the next generation of advocates for family-centred service.

In a truly family-centred environment, service providers, families and individuals will realize that family-centred service is never fully achieved– it is a journey that will continue as long as families' and individuals' needs continue to change.

REFERENCES

1. Murphy DL, Lee IM. *Family-Centered Program Rating Scale: User's Manual, ed 2.* Lawrence, KS: Beach Center on Families and Disability, The University of Kansas; 1991.

2. Dunst C, Johanson C, Trivette C, Hamby D. Family oriented early intervention policies and practices: family-centered or not? *Except Child.* 1991; 21(11): 115-118.

3. Draper N. *Delivering Services for Children with Special Needs and Their Families: A Collaborative Approach.* Willowdale, Ontario: Bloorview MacMillan Centre; 1996.

4. Shelton T, Stepenek JS. *Family-Centered Care for Children Needing Specialized Health and Developmental Services.* Bethesda, MD: Association for the Care of Children's Health (ACCH); 1994.

5. Friesen B, Koroloff N. Family-centred services: implications for mental health administration and research. *J Mental Health Admin.* 1990; 17(1):13-25.

6. Birkmeier K. Nurturing and empowering the family. *NDTA Network.* 1994; July: 7.

Occupational Performance Needs
of School-Aged Children
with Physical Disabilities
in the Community

Nancy Pollock
Debra Stewart

SUMMARY. Over the past several years major shifts have occurred in the delivery of therapy services to children with physical disabilities. Services have moved from centre- or clinic-based to school-

Nancy Pollock, MSc, OT(C), is Assistant Clinical Professor, School of Rehabilitation Science and Co-Investigator, Neurodevelopmental Clinical Research Unit, McMaster University, Hamilton, ON. Debra Stewart, BSc, OT(C), is Occupational Therapist, Erinoak, Serving Young People with Physical Disabilities, Mississauga, ON, and Clinical Lecturer, School of Rehabilitation Science, McMaster University.

Address correspondence to: Nancy Pollock, School of Rehabilitation Science, McMaster University, Building T-16, 1280 Main Street West, Hamilton, ON, Canada L8S 4K1.

The authors wish to acknowledge the support and efforts of the children, families, and occupational therapists affiliated with Erinoak, Serving Young People with Physical Disabilities, in Mississauga, ON, the Children's Developmental Rehabilitation Program in Hamilton, ON, and the teachers and educational assistants who participated. The authors also wish to thank Debra Cameron, Deb Agro, Qin Lu, Leanne LeClair and Thomas Morrison for their assistance in the completion of this project.

This project was funded by a grant from the Canadian Occupational Therapy Foundation.

[Haworth co-indexing entry note]: "Occupational Performance Needs of School-Aged Children with Physical Disabilities in the Community." Pollock, Nancy, and Debra Stewart. Co-published simultaneously in *Physical & Occupational Therapy in Pediatrics* (The Haworth Press, Inc.) Vol. 18, No. 1, 1998, pp. 55-68; and: *Family-Centred Assessment and Intervention in Pediatric Rehabilitation* (ed: Mary Law) The Haworth Press, Inc., 1998, pp. 55-68. Single or multiple copies of this article are available for a fee from The Haworth Document Delivery Service [1-800-342-9678, 9:00 a.m. - 5:00 p.m. (EST). E-mail address: getinfo@ haworthpressinc.com].

based. Direct care has been supplemented by consultation, and an adaptive model has superseded more traditional remedial approaches. These shifts appear to have been made largely in response to system changes, fiscal constraints and the integration of more students with special needs into the mainstream of education. The changes do not appear to have been driven by client need, but rather therapist and system needs.

The purpose of this study was to increase our understanding of the occupational performance needs of young school-aged children with physical disabilities in the school system and the community, and to identify how therapists can help to meet those needs. Using the Canadian Occupational Performance Measure, 202 parents, teachers and children were interviewed, and their top priority problems were identified. In-depth interviews with 18 parents and teachers provided additional information about needs, ideas for change, and the role that therapists can play in meeting those needs.

The results of this study provide some clear directions for service delivery planning and suggest that the recent trends in practice, although not originally derived from client needs, will support the families and schools in meeting the needs of the children. *[Article copies available for a fee from The Haworth Document Delivery Service: 1-800-342-9678. E-mail address: getinfo@haworthpressinc.com]*

Therapy services for school-aged children with disabilities have changed dramatically over the past two decades in location of service, methods of delivery and focus of the therapy. Occupational therapists and physical therapists have moved from institutional settings such as clinics and treatment centres to the community, in particular the child's school.[1,2] Practice in these natural settings allows for the therapy to be more relevant to the daily lives of the children.[3,4] Service delivery models have also shifted from primarily direct service to include more consultative models.[5,6] Therapists are working with teachers and other education personnel to collaborate in goal setting, program planning and intervention to meet students' needs. The focus of therapy has also changed from a strong emphasis on the remediation of performance component deficits to one of compensation or adaptation to allow the child to perform more successfully, not more normally, in the school setting.[7]

These changes in practice have come in response to a number of societal changes: legislation, increased inclusion of children with special needs in mainstream education, increased demand for services, and fiscal constraints.[8] Although many of the forces of change are positive ones, some are not. Increasing caseloads and decreasing resources are a reality in most jurisdictions today and are likely behind some of the service delivery changes we have seen in recent years. Although constraints can sometimes lead to positive innovations, a risk is that clients' needs will not be met. This concern led us to question whether changes we had made in our practice were good ones from the perspective of the clients we serve. If we are client-centred service providers, then our service must be determined by client needs, not program mandates, caseload demands or institutional policies.

The main purpose of this study was to increase our understanding of the occupational performance needs of young school-aged children with physical disabilities in the school system and community, and to identify how therapists can help to meet those needs from a client/caregiver perspective. As Bundy states . . .

> Therapists are service providers; their job is infinitely more difficult when they attempt to determine the direction of a student's intervention without the active involvement of the student and his or her parents and teachers.[9(p 8)]

Specific objectives were:

1. to assess a group of children with physical disabilities, their parents and their teachers using the Canadian Occupational Performance Measure (COPM) to understand the occupational performance needs of the children;
2. to interview a sub-sample of parents and teachers to explore further their perceptions of the children's needs and the role that therapists can play in meeting those needs;
3. to examine the identified occupational performance needs for commonality and developmental trends; and
4. to make recommendations on service delivery in the community, including the school system, for children with physical disabilities.

METHODS

Occupational therapists from teams serving school-aged clients at two children's treatment centres in Ontario, Canada, agreed to participate in the study and acted as the primary data gatherers. Children with physical disabilities in the regular school system between kindergarten and grade four were eligible for the study. The occupational therapists identified potential subjects from their existing caseloads and sought consent from parents and teachers. They then completed a COPM with the parents and teachers and, where possible, with the children themselves.

From the total sample, a sub-group of parents and teachers was randomly selected for an interview. Half of the interviews were conducted before the COPM and half after to balance the potential effects of testing on the interview. The focus of this interview was to explore in a less structured way the clients' needs, expectations of therapy and perceptions of the COPM process. The interviews were conducted by an independent interviewer (research assistant) unaware of the results of the COPM. Interviews were audiotaped and transcribed for analysis.

Sample

The final sample included 92 children. Of the 92 subjects, all had a parent and a teacher participating in completion of the COPM, and in 18 cases, the child was also included as a respondent for a total of 202 COPMs. Interviews were completed with 18 respondents, 9 teachers and 9 parents. Table 1 describes the sample in more detail.

Measurement

The Canadian Occupational Performance Measure was the primary measure used. The COPM[10] was designed to operationalize the Guidelines for the Client-centred Practice of Occupational Therapy.[11] It allows the client to identify the areas of occupational performance that present them with problems and to prioritize those concerns. The scoring yields a performance and a satisfaction score. The COPM is not diagnosis-specific, can be used across all developmental ages, and can be given to caregivers as well as to clients. A training session was held with all the participating therapists and on-going support was given by the investigators throughout the study.

For the in-depth interviews, the questions were developed by the investigators, pre-tested on two clients and then revised. The questions were fairly open-ended to allow the interviewees to give a broad range of answers and comments.

The four questions and subsequent probes were:

1. What do you see as your child's/this student's needs at this point in time (probe for different contexts, e.g., school, home, community)?
2. As occupational therapists, we believe it's important to have a balance between work, self-care, play and rest. How well do you feel your child/this student is achieving that balance?
3. What changes would you like to see happen to meet some of the needs you have talked about (probe for different contexts, i.e., changes in the child, the home, the school, the community)?
4. How do you feel therapists can contribute to those changes?

TABLE 1. Description of Study Sample

	%
Gender	
female	41.3
male	58.7
Grade Level	
kindergarten	20.7
grade one	19.6
grade two	17.4
grade three	13.0
grade four	15.2
special class	14.1
Diagnosis	
cerebral palsy	35.9
spina bifida	15.2
developmental delay	9.8
Williams syndrome	3.3
other*	35.8
Functional Mobility	
walks unaided	52.2
uses crutches	3.3
uses walker	6.5
uses manual chair	28.2
uses power chair	9.8
Communication	
verbal	78.0
augmentative	9.9
other**	11.0
Assistance Required in Activities of Daily Living	
total	20.7
considerable	16.3
moderate	32.6
slight	23.9
none	6.5

*   other diagnoses include 24 different conditions
** other communication includes sign, gesture or no communication

Analysis

The data analysis included a number of different approaches and steps. Each therapist completed a demographic profile of the subjects. Descriptive statistics were generated from these profiles. The COPM results were coded for type of problem and entered into a database package and analyzed. The coding scheme represents the problems identified by the respondents and was developed through a consensus process. The investigators developed an initial coding scheme from 30 completed COPMs. They then met with a research assistant to code an additional 15 COPMs and reach agreement on the codes. The research assistant then completed the rest of the coding.

The interview transcripts were analyzed using a descriptive method. They were read repeatedly and discussed by the investigators and the research assistant to extract common issues and ideas that were identified by the respondents in relation to client needs and the role of the therapist in meeting those needs.

COPM RESULTS

As shown in Table 1, the age spread of the subjects was fairly even across the grade levels, and children with a wide variety of diagnoses were included in the sample. The majority of children were independently mobile, but most required some level of assistance to complete their activities of daily living.

The final code list of problems identified from the COPM contained over 1700 items. For the purpose of analysis, these items were collapsed down to 35 categories representing areas of occupational performance in self-care, productivity and leisure. Only those items that were rated as priorities (maximum 5 per respondent) have been included in the results.

The problems identified most frequently (i.e., those mentioned by more than 20% of the respondents) by the teachers, parents and children are listed in Table 2. Although 18 children were interviewed using the COPM, only 10 were able to prioritize the problem areas. One teacher was unable to identify any problems. Overall, most parents, teachers, and children identified mobility as their greatest area of concern.

Another of our research questions was to determine how often the parents and teachers agreed on the priority problems. Figure 1 shows the level of agreement between parents and teachers. Most agreed on one or two problems out of a possible five.

The results were examined to detect any developmental trends, i.e., do issues differ based on the age of the child? Trends were present but were

TABLE 2. Priority Problems from COPM

	%
Parents (n = 92)	
mobility	58.7
dressing	54.3
toileting	43.5
socialization	33.7
hygiene	27.2
written work	27.2
play	21.7
Teachers (n = 91)	
mobility	63.2
behavior	54.0
socialization	47.8
dressing	46.0
play	27.6
toileting	27.6
written work	26.4
Children (n = 10)	
mobility	90.0
active leisure	60.0
written work	40.0
bathing	30.0
school activities	30.0
academics	30.0

quite weak in this sample. Overall, self-care issues became less of a concern for older children. Issues around behavior and socialization increased in prominence for children in the higher grade levels. Mobility remained as the highest priority problem across the age range.

We also searched for any relationships between the severity of the child's disability and the type of problems identified. No differences in the type of problem identified were found, but, overall, the children who were more independent or higher functioning were identified as having a greater number of problems than those who were more severely involved.

INTERVIEW RESULTS

One of the objectives of the interviews was to compare the types of needs identified through the COPM to the needs identified in a more

FIGURE 1. Agreement

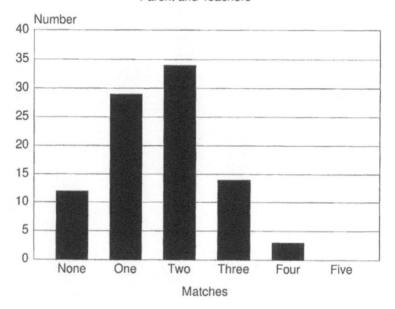

Parent and Teachers

Matches

open-ended interview. Eighteen interviews were conducted–9 with parents and 9 with teaching staff (7 classroom teachers, 1 resource teacher and 1 teaching assistant). Table 3 describes the problem areas most frequently described during the interviews. The areas identified are very similar to those identified during the COPM, although the frequencies are different. Issues around communication and active leisure, specifically access to community recreation programs, came up on the interviews more than on the COPM. Figure 2 shows the level of agreement between the problems identified through the COPM and those identified through the interview. The majority of respondents agreed on two or three problem areas between the two methods.

What is perhaps more interesting when comparing the COPM and interview results are the differences, i.e., those needs that were identified through the COPM but not during the interview and vice versa. It is apparent that the two methods of assessment elicit different information. The responses on the COPM were child focused, i.e., identified problems the child was encountering within his or her environment. The interviews tended to reveal "other" issues that related more to the respondent (i.e.,

TABLE 3. Priority Problems from Interviews

	%
Parents (n = 9)	
mobility	44
socialization	44
active leisure	44
eating	33
dressing	33
written work	33
computer	33
toileting	22
behavior	22
Teachers (n = 9)	
communications	44
toileting	44
written work	33
eating	22
behavior	22
computer	22

FIGURE 2. Agreement

COPM and Interview (n = 18)

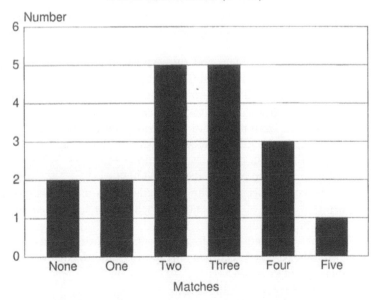

the concerns or needs of the parent or teacher) or to a "system" including the school system and community services.

As part of the analysis of the interview results, the interviews that were conducted prior to the COPM were compared to those interviews done after the COPM. Some differences were found in the respondents' answers, as agreement between the COPM and interview-identified needs was slightly higher on the post-COPM interviews (44% agreement on post-COPM interviews versus 34% agreement on pre-COPM interviews). Although completing the COPM appeared to have some effect on the answers a respondent gave during the interview, the small sample makes drawing any conclusions difficult.

A second objective of the interviews was to explore the respondents' perceptions and expectations of therapists. Many parents and teachers spoke of the dilemmas they face on a daily basis in caring for or teaching a child with a physical disability. They were often uncertain if their expectations were appropriate and didn't feel they had adequate information to make informed decisions or adaptations. The respondents offered some interesting perspectives on the role and functions of therapists when they work with children/students and their parents and teachers. Their ideas are probably relevant to all therapists and clinicians.

Some of the recurring messages from the respondents were:

1. Change the environment, not the child. Focus on adapting the environment and the activity so that the child can be more successful, not more normal. Don't invest your energies in trying to "fix" the child.
2. Incorporate your ideas and suggestions into our daily routines and activities. Make them practical and easy to accomplish.
3. Individualize your programs. Recognize our individuality and offer flexible programs that allow us to select options or make choices.
4. Prepare us. Help us to plan ahead, to think of issues that we might be facing in the future but are unaware of at present.
5. Support us in our decisions, our actions, our ideas. Tell us when we are doing a good job or have a good idea.
6. Share your ideas and your knowledge with us. As therapists you bring a wealth of experience to each of our individual situations. Share that wealth.
7. Educate us about child development, about disabilities and about systems. We need adequate and appropriate information in order to make good decisions.

8. Communicate with us. Keep us informed about what you're doing and help us to be part of the team. You can facilitate communication between home and school.
9. Network with us and facilitate opportunities for us to network with each other.
10. Advocate on our behalf. Work with us to advocate for more/better services, for improved access to services, for flexibility in the services offered, and help us to cut through the red tape.

DISCUSSION

The needs of the children with disabilities. We have learned a great deal from listening to our clients using both the COPM and the interviews. The COPM has shown us the problems occurring most frequently for children in this sample. Issues around mobility, self-care, written work, and play were commonly raised by both teachers and parents. Teachers were more concerned than parents about behavior at school and socialization. This may be due to the environment the child is in and the expectations within that setting. School is typically more structured than home and there are many more demands for cooperation, concentration and self-organization. Teachers also see the children consistently in a group with their peers where they observe how the child interacts with his or her peers. Parents would have fewer opportunities to see the child with their peers. Not surprisingly, parents rated toileting as a priority more frequently than teachers. The role of toileting a child with special needs typically falls to the educational assistant at school so teachers would be less familiar with the concerns.

The children in this sample appeared to present with fairly consistent problems from kindergarten to grade four. No strong developmental trends were noted. This is important information when considering service planning. The children with less severe disabilities appeared to have a greater number of problems. Although this may seem surprising, it is often a reflection of the higher expectations placed on the children who appear more normal. Also, by this age, most families will have put systems and strategies in place to care for a child with severe disabilities.

Service delivery and the role of the therapists. Parents and teachers appeared to value the involvement of therapists and were able to articulate clearly where they believe therapists could have an impact. Of interest was that only two of the eighteen respondents wanted more direct "hands-on" intervention for the child from the therapist. The rest focused on more indirect roles for the therapist including consultation, mediator training and advocacy. The impetus for this study was to determine how the changes being made in service delivery were affecting our ability to meet our clients' needs. The results of this study support that the changes made have been positive changes.

Support is also provided for the changes in the focus of our intervention. As occupational therapists we have moved to more of an adaptive philosophy than a remedial philosophy with this age group of children. Rather than concentrating on trying to change the child's abilities or skills, we have put more emphasis on trying to adapt the environment around the child and the activities in which the child is engaged. This philosophy was strongly supported, particularly by parents.

The results support our shift to a community-based focus for our services, in particular our emphasis on school-based service. Parents and teachers emphasized the need for therapists to incorporate ideas and suggestions into the child's daily routine. In order to understand that routine, and the specifics of the child's environment, therapists need to be in the environments where the child is functioning on a daily basis. Also, with the increased emphasis on adapting the environment around the child, therapy needs to occur in the natural settings to be able to make changes in the physical and social environments. The participants also spoke about the need to network and to facilitate communication among the team members working with the child and family. If therapy occurs in a more isolated setting such as a clinic, this type of teamwork is very difficult to achieve.

Another shift has been to offer less direct intervention to the child and more consultation and mediator training to those around the child to help them maximize the child's function. Parents and teachers spoke about their need for education, information, support, resources and advocacy, all functions that can best be accomplished through working collaboratively with caregivers. For many therapists trained with an emphasis on one-to-one interaction and intervention with children, consultation and mediator training are often less comfortable roles and are frequently perceived to be of less value than direct treatment. It is heartening to see that in fact this is what our clients are asking for. These results support the need for the continuation of professional education focused on collaboration, consultation and the skills necessary for effective community practice.

Family/client-centred practice. The respondents in this study reinforced our ideas about client-centred practice. We need to consider the individual in every interaction and in planning our service. Every individual we spoke to had different ideas, thoughts, needs, dilemmas, coping abilities and priorities. They all require flexible, individualized services. They also require information and support to help them make decisions to meet their own needs. This study reinforced the need to broaden our view of the client to include parents, siblings, teachers, respite workers, extended families, educational assistants, community agencies, and school boards. Our involvement needs to extend beyond the child to include those in the child's environment.

Finally, our clients told us about the need to work collaboratively with each other, to communicate effectively and to coordinate our services. They believe that therapists have a role in fostering partnerships and facilitating that collaboration. They believe that through our holistic approach to our clients we can bring together the child, the family, the school and the broader community to work together in the best interests of all concerned.

LIMITATIONS AND FUTURE DIRECTIONS

Although this sample was representative of the population served by these children's treatment centres, it may not be representative of the broader population. We tried to ensure broad representation of ages and disability levels and therefore did not use a random selection method. This purposeful sampling may have introduced an inclusion bias. The therapists selected the subjects and may, therefore, have excluded families they believe would have difficulty doing the COPM. These families may well have identified different issues, again limiting the generalizability of the results.

This study was conducted by occupational therapists and, as a result, focused on the domain of occupation. Many of the issues raised by families and teachers, however, are relevant to other clinicians working with this population.

As with most research, this study has generated more questions than it has answered. Some of our immediate plans are to do secondary analyses of the data to look more closely at the complete range of problems identified, not just the prioritized ones. We want to investigate differences between the problems the therapists anticipated would be identified prior to administration of the COPM and the ones the parents and teachers actually identified. We plan to interview the participating therapists to understand how, why and when they are choosing to use the COPM in their practice.

In the longer term it would be most interesting to do a similar study with older students to examine the changing needs as the children age. A higher percentage of older children would be able to respond to the COPM themselves and would provide a valuable perspective.

REFERENCES

1. American Occupational Therapy Association: *Membership survey data report*, 1995. Bethesda, MD: Author; 1995.

2. Canadian Association of Occupational Therapists: *Membership profile*, 1995. Ottawa, ON: Author; 1995.

3. Dunn W, Brown C, McGuigan A: The ecology of human performance: a framework for considering the impact of context. *Am J Occup Ther.* 1994; 48: 595-607.

4. McEwen IR, Shelden ML: Pediatric therapy in the 1990s: the demise of the educational versus medical dichotomy. *Phys Occup Ther Pediatr.* 1995; 15(2): 33-45.

5. Case-Smith J, Cable J: Perceptions of occupational therapists regarding service delivery models in school-based practice. *Occ Ther J Res.* 1996; 16:23-44.

6. Kemmis BL, Dunn W: Collaborative consultation: the efficacy of remedial and compensatory interventions in school contexts. *Am J Occup Ther.* 1996; 50: 709-717.

7. Rourk JD: Roles for school-based occupational therapists: Past, present, future. *Am J Occup Ther.* 1996; 50:698-700.

8. Johnson J: School-based occupational therapy. In: Case-Smith J, Allen AS, Clark PN, eds. *Occupational Therapy for Children*. St. Louis, MO: Mosby; 1996: 693-716.

9. Bundy AC: *Making a Difference: OTs and PTs in Public Schools. A Model Curriculum for Preparing Occupational and Physical Therapy Students to Practice in Schools*. Chicago, IL: University of Illinois at Chicago; 1991.

10. Law M, Baptiste S, Carswell A, McColl M, Polatajko H, Pollock N: *COPM (2nd ed.)*. Toronto: CAOT Publications ACE; 1994.

11. Canadian Association of Occupational Therapists: *Occupational Therapy Guidelines for Client-centred Practice*. Ottawa: CAOT Publications; 1991.

Planning Rehabilitation:
A Comparison of Issues
for Parents and Adolescents

Heather McGavin

SUMMARY. Therapists often question who the client is when dealing with adolescents and their parents. A cross-sectional survey was done with 14 families to determine how rehabilitation goals differ between parents and adolescents. The Canadian Occupational Performance Measure was administered to each adolescent and parent(s). Parents identified 261 issues and adolescents identified 138 with an 8.77% level of agreement. Priorities were determined and the percentage of agreement was 10.94%. The results of this survey support clinicians' reports about discrepancies between parents' and adolescents' rehabilitation goals and warrant further exploration. The development of strategies for including adolescents in the rehabilitation partnership is recommended. *[Article copies available for a fee from The Haworth Document Delivery Service: 1-800-342-9678. E-mail address: getinfo@haworthpressinc.com]*

Heather McGavin, MHSc, is Physiotherapist, Hamilton Health Sciences Corporation (Chedoke-McMaster Division) and part-time Clinical Lecturer, School of Rehabilitation Science, McMaster University, Hamilton, ON.

Address correspondence to: Heather McGavin, Children's Developmental Rehabilitation Programme, Hamilton Health Sciences Corporation, Chedoke Site, Box 2000, Hamilton, ON, Canada L8N 3Z5.

The author would like to acknowledge the support of the Neurodevelopmental Clinical Research Unit, Hamilton, ON, and Mary Law, PhD, OT(C), who served as advisor for this project.

[Haworth co-indexing entry note]: "Planning Rehabilitation: A Comparison of Issues for Parents and Adolescents." McGavin, Heather. Co-published simultaneously in *Physical & Occupational Therapy in Pediatrics* (The Haworth Press, Inc.) Vol. 18, No. 1, 1998, pp. 69-82; and: *Family-Centred Assessment and Intervention in Pediatric Rehabilitation* (ed: Mary Law) The Haworth Press, Inc., 1998, pp. 69-82. Single or multiple copies of this article are available for a fee from The Haworth Document Delivery Service [1-800-342-9678, 9:00 a.m. - 5:00 p.m. (EST). E-mail address: getinfo@haworthpressinc.com].

INTRODUCTION

In paediatric rehabilitation, a family-centred service delivery model is becoming widely adopted.[1-5] One of the challenges in providing family-centred service is the difficulty of working with more than one client, e.g., the adolescent *and* the parents. Adolescents' goals may differ from those of their parents. The literature on family-centredness, largely developed with pre-school services, does not give service providers direction with how to deal with this dilemma.

LITERATURE REVIEW

Family-Centred Service

The origins of family-centred service go back to Carl Rogers who founded the school of "Client-Centered Therapy" in the 1940's.[6] Its principles fostered personal growth and development and a re-direction of therapy towards what was meaningful to the client. During the last 20 years, a growing realization has been that parents know their children better than anyone else, and they have become more active participants in the rehabilitation process.[7,8]

Family-centered care has many definitions. It is, according to Bailey, McWilliam, and Winton, "a concept based on basic values and philosophic assumptions."[2(p 74)] Its basic tenets include empowerment, collaboration, informed decision making, a recognition that the family is the constant in a child's life, the availability of support and networking, and a respect for families' cultural diversities and methods of coping.[5]

The shift to family-centred service has not been an easy one. In 1984 Cadman, Goldsmith, and Bashim[9] determined that values and preferences do not always match between professionals and families. This discrepancy of values has necessitated more negotiating and flexibility on the part of health care professionals.[1,10] To be family-centred, service providers' competencies must now include empathetic listening, consulting, teaching, enabling, advocacy, and mediating.[10] A greater knowledge of family systems, coping methods, cultural beliefs and values[3,11] and a belief in the rights of parents are intrinsic to the success of family-centred service.

Adolescence

Adolescence is a journey of personal growth and the establishment of self-identity which requires the evaluating and critiquing of adult values and a determination of their applicability to oneself.[12] It is a time of withdrawal from adults and of forming allegiances with peers. Peer groups provide a social arena for experimentation with new roles within a supportive environment, a sense of belonging, and social interaction. Two authors have summarized Erikson's formulations about adolescence and have stated that the tasks of adolescence are to: (1) establish identity and self-image, (2) move away from family, (3) establish an adult sexual role, and (4) make career and vocational choices.[13,14] Accomplishing these tasks is difficult for many adolescents with disabilities. They are often rejected by their peers,[15] and, physically, many are not capable of withdrawing from adults. Their most valuable resource of a peer group is not available to them on their journey of personal growth. Self-perception is a key element in the development of self-identity, and, therefore, to capture what adolescents perceive to be the key issues in their lives is important, particularly if their perceptions are different from their parents' views.

METHOD

The purpose of the study was to answer the question "How do rehabilitation issues compare between parents and adolescents?" A cross-sectional survey of a sample of clients from a children's rehabilitation service was done. Study participants were adolescents between the ages of 13 and 19 years, with a diagnosis of some type of physical disability and enough verbal skills to express basic needs adequately.

A group of 103 adolescents was identified, but after their communication status was reviewed, 67 adolescents were eligible. Further exclusions included 2 for personal reasons, one family who did not speak English, and 2 because they were on the researcher's own case load. This left 62 adolescents. A letter was sent out to each of the families by the Programme Manager explaining the study and inviting them to participate. Fourteen families agreed to participate.

OUTCOME MEASURE

The Canadian Occupational Performance Measure (COPM)[16] was designed to assess client outcomes in various performance areas and is based on the Model of Occupational Performance.[17] The Model of Occupational Performance provides a framework that addresses tasks and activities within an individual's own environment, and the COPM is an individualized measure that is based on one's own perceptions about occupational performance. It provides a framework from which to explore all aspects of an individual's daily activities and the perceived issues and concerns that arise from performance in self-care, productivity and leisure activities. It allows clients to evaluate their performance and determine how satisfied they are with it. The COPM focuses on clients' issues within their own environment and addresses their unique perspectives and priorities. For young children, or those incapable of responding, caregivers can provide their perspective and identify concerns. Therapeutic goals are determined on the basis of the most important issues identified. The COPM can be used at any stage in life and is well suited for use with adolescents.

The COPM is a tool that can be used with any disability group. It is administered through an interview process in which the client identifies issues or concerns regarding various activities in daily life that he or she wants to do, needs to do, or is expected to do. Performance is addressed within the three aforementioned domains of self-care, productivity and leisure. Self-care incorporates personal care, functional mobility and community management, while productivity addresses paid/unpaid work, household management and play/school activities. Leisure activities include quiet and active recreation as well as socialization. Probing questions are often required for purposes of clarification.

Once issues have been identified, the client is asked to rate the activities in terms of importance to his or her life. A ten-point scale is used with the rating of 1 being "not important at all" and a rating of 10 being "extremely important." The client is then asked to choose the five problems that are the most important. Usually the items with the highest importance ratings are chosen. For each of these five items, the client is then asked to rate his or her performance for this activity. Again, a ten-point scale is used with a score of 1 being "not able to do it at all" and a score of 10 being "able to do it extremely well." Finally, the client is asked to rate his or her satisfaction with how well he or she performs the activity, again using a 10-point scale. The range is from "not satisfied at all" to "extremely satisfied." Mean scores across activities for both performance and satisfaction are calculated. For the purposes of this study, the initial scores were used for comparison between parents and adolescents. The COPM has been shown to be sensitive to change and has good test-retest reliability.[16]

RESULTS

The average age of the adolescents was 15.5 years (SD = 2.06). Grades ranged from grade 7 to 13. Seven of the students were receiving modified educational programming. Diagnoses and other family demographic data can be found in Table 1.

Twenty-eight interviews were completed in total, 14 with parents and 14 with adolescents. Eleven of the parent interviews were with mothers only. One was with the father only, and two of the interviews were with both parents. Twenty-four of the 28 interviews were in the families' homes. One was held at the adolescent's school, one was held at the mother's place of employment, and two interviews were held at the reha-

TABLE 1. Demographic Data on Subjects

Diagnoses of adolescents

Acquired Brain Injury	1
Alternating Hemiplegia of Childhood	1
Cerebral Palsy	9
Spina Bifida & Hydrocephalus	2
Spinal Cord Injury	1

Ages of adolescents

13 years	3
14 years	3
15 years	2
16 years	1
17 years	1
18 years	3
19 years	1

Academic status of adolescents

Grade 7	2
Grade 8	1
Grade 9	3
Grade 10	3
Grade 11	1
Grade 12	3
Grade 13	1
Those receiving modified programming	7

Parental respondents

Mother only	11
Father only	1
Mother and Father	2

Adolescent respondents

Male	6
Female	8

Marital status of parents

Married	11
Single parent	2
Common-law	1

Average age of parents (years)

Mothers	42
Fathers	44

Extended family

nearby	9
nearby & described as close	1
nearby but not much support	1
minimal involvement	1
none nearby	2

Employment

Mothers - outside the home		9
	self-employed	1
	homemakers	4
Fathers - employed or self-employed		11
	unemployed	1

bilitation centre. The adolescents' interviews averaged 27 minutes in length, while parental interviews averaged 61 minutes.

Self-Care

One of the areas that raised the greatest number of concerns for the parents was self-care. The assistance and supervision required was of concern because of the implications for future independence. Adolescents mentioned these concerns also, but to a lesser degree. Parents identified frustration with the constant reminding in which they engage because of the adolescents' lack of interest in personal grooming and hygiene.

A similar number of issues were identified by parents and adolescents in the areas of transfers and ambulation, but the focus varied. Adolescents were more concerned about tub and shower transfers, and the parents were more concerned about the difficulty that their sons and daughters have transferring in and out of vehicles. Nine out of the 14 adolescents use wheelchairs and several parents expressed concern that they were walking less than previously. The adolescents indicated difficulties with endurance, stability, and safety outdoors when walking. None of the adolescents were driving yet, but it was a concern to parents whose adolescents had expressed an interest in it.

Discussions about managing in the community brought out concerns about transportation and accessibility, but the main issues of concern related to management of money. Several of the adolescents identified their difficulties in handling money. Parents identified this issue also, but were mainly concerned about others taking advantage of their children.

Productivity

Parents believed that the potential for paying jobs was limited because of their adolescents' disabilities. Only one adolescent indicated that she was concerned about job refusal because of her disability while two adolescents expressed concern about their lack of work experience.

Household management, particularly kitchen-based activities, is an area of frustration for both parents and adolescents. Both parents and adolescents mentioned that assistance was required for many activities. Some adolescents indicated that they would like to be able to do more chores around the house, but parents expressed frustration about finding tasks that their adolescents could do independently.

Parents' concerns outweighed the adolescents' in the area of school and were related to problems at school and adolescents' attitudes towards school. The adolescents identified academic problems as well as problems related to personal time organization, having few friends at school, and being treated like children.

Leisure

Parents had many concerns about quiet recreational pursuits (too much time indoors, alone, and limited reading skills). They believed that their adolescents were not active enough and were choosing sedentary activities. The adolescents made little mention of these concerns, but they did have concerns about active recreation and sports. They wanted more availability of "disabled" sports activities and they wanted to be able to play sports better. Socialization was a source of great concern to most participants. Several adolescents and their parents indicated that the adolescents had few friends, and a few indicated that they do not do much with friends. Only one young lady was satisfied with her friends. Limited involvement with peers was of concern to several of the parents and concern about peer influence was also mentioned by three parents and one adolescent.

Relationship issues were of concern to many parents. Almost half of the parents believed that their sons' and daughters' social skills were limited. Some concerns were expressed about the motives of individuals developing relationships with their children and the potential for their daughters to be taken advantage of in relationships.

Other Issues

Many parents mentioned general issues of concern not directly related to issues on the COPM. Concern about the future was expressed by most parents. They want their sons and daughters to be contributing members of society but are unsure about jobs and living arrangements. They would like their adolescents to be independent but were discouraged about the realities of the situations that they were facing. Several of the adolescents stated that they wanted to get out and live on their own. The other major issue mentioned by over half of the parents was that of the vulnerability of their adolescents (mainly daughters). They had concerns about their vulnerability physically, socially, and financially. One set of parents expressed concern about the impact of having a child with a disability on his or her siblings.

Summary

Parents and adolescents agreed upon few issues. A summary of the issues identified can be found in Table 2. Parents identified a total of 261

TABLE 2. Issues Identified by Parents and Adolescents

	Number of times identified	
	Parents	Adolescents
Self-Care		
Personal Care		
Hygiene/bathing/grooming	26	12
Dressing	9	6
Eating	5	3
Drooling	1	
Weight	1	1
Functional Mobility		
Transfers	10	9
Ambulation	15	10
Wheelchair use	3	5
Driving	3	2
Bike riding		1
Community Management		
Finances	9	4
Transportation	4	4
Accessibility		2
Initiative	4	1
Problem-solving with tasks	1	
Vulnerability	4	
Productivity		
Paid/Unpaid Work		
Jobs	13	4
Volunteering	3	2
Household Management		
Chores	11	7
Kitchen	8	
Concepts	4	3
Homework	3	3
Computer use	1	
Written work	2	1
Supports	2	2
Problems	7	3
Adolescents' attitudes	8	2
Leisure		
Quiet Recreation		
T.V.	3	1
Leisure time	6	1
Activities	4	1
Limitations	3	

| | Number of times identified | |
	Parents	Adolescents
Active Recreation		
Sports	7	16
Exercise/fitness	4	
Camp		1
Travel		1
Outdoor activities	9	2
Accessibility	4	
Miscellaneous	5	2
Social		
Friends	11	7
Peers	8	2
Relationships	11	3
Families	2	
Social situations	8	2
Other issues	42	5

issues and the adolescents identified 138. Among these were 35 similar issues, for an agreement of 8.77% between parents and adolescents. For those issues, the importance ratings were compared. Fourteen were in exact agreement, 7 had a 1-2 point difference, and 14 had > 2 points difference.

Each adolescent and parent was asked to identify five priority issues. All of the parents listed five priorities, but the number of priorities for adolescents ranged from one to five. The priority ratings of the five most important issues were compared. Eight families had no agreement. Five families had agreement on one priority, and one family had agreement on two priorities. This gave an overall percentage of agreement of 10.94%.

For the seven agreed upon priorities, the performance and satisfaction ratings were also compared. For the performance ratings, one was in exact agreement, three had a 1-3 point difference, and three had > 2 points difference. For the satisfaction ratings, four were in exact agreement, two had a 1-2 point difference, and one had > 2 points difference.

DISCUSSION

The purpose of this study was to determine how adolescents' issues for rehabilitation compared to issues identified by their parents. With a level of agreement between issues of 8.77%, the issues appear to be very different with this particular group; however, this answer alone is not enough. One must then ask "in what way are they different?"

Considering the large number of issues related to self-care, parents clearly still feel responsible for their sons' or daughters' personal care. Dependency for self-care by adolescents with disabilities is common[15,18-20] and can have negative implications for both parents and adolescents. Although only the parents had issues about the need for reminders about personal care, almost as many adolescents as parents were concerned about the assistance required from their parents. They are bothered that they still require help doing simple tasks such as washing hair, getting in and out of the tub, doing up buttons, or putting on socks. They do not want to be dependent on their parents for these tasks but, for the most part, they were accepting of the fact that they require assistance. As one young man in the study indicated, "Needing help is a reality of life." Several authors[15,19,21,22] have reported that adolescents with disabilities are significantly lower in their independence than able-bodied adolescents, and other authors[14,15,23,24] have discussed many negative aspects of this dependency. Independence was the ultimate goal for several of the adolescents in the study and most of the parents want this also. The parents are often realistic and discouraged about the difficulties in achieving independence, while the adolescents believe that it is possible.

Desired independence was also affected by the adolescents' mobility skills. The concerns about the use of crutches, walkers, and wheelchairs all related to the adolescents' desire to manage on their own. The adolescents' limited mobility, as well as their physical skills, affected their recreational pursuits. All of the adolescents interviewed rely on sports activities that are organized for youth with disabilities. Many believe that the options for them in this area are limited. A desire to become more involved and more skilled was a major issue with many of them. This agrees with the findings of King et al.[19] and Hansen[25] who found that both male and female adolescents with physical disabilities perceived that they had lowered athletic competence.

Parents were less concerned with competence, however, than with general activity levels and choices of activities and these concerns are well supported in the literature.[14,20,25,26] They would like their adolescents to be more active and involved. How much of the passive activity observed with this population is a part of the inherent nature of the individuals and how much is generated by their own environment is unknown. Looking broadly at general recreational activities, Skrtic, Summers, Brotherson, and Turnbull[27] have mentioned that recreational activities in the community were often limited by accessibility and opportunity—an issue raised more than once by the parents in this study.

Besides the concerns about self-care, the most predominant issue that was raised during these interviews related to social life. For many adolescents, the current situation was unsatisfactory. They want to spend more time with their peers and have closer friendships. The parents shared these concerns but their concerns were also about friendship requirements–addressing interaction skills and looking at personal attributes that affect relationships. These concerns are well supported and are discussed by many different authors. Concerns raised about social skills and relationships have validity.[13,22,24,28-30] These adolescents may be missing some valuable opportunities to facilitate moving on to adulthood.

Some authors have studied factors related to the social development of individuals. Strax[14] and Blum et al.[18] both discuss the effect of mobility limitations for these individuals. Strax also indicated that adolescents with disabilities are often rejected, and that this in itself leads to the use of inappropriate behaviour in efforts to find friends. Other authors[21,24-26,31,32] refer to the limited social interactions available to adolescents with disabilities.

Concern about the future is another part of the mosaic that makes up the world of adolescents with disabilities and their parents. Physically, these adolescents are restricted from some jobs and many of them have no experience to support them when looking for employment. Often, those with disabilities are expected to have more experience than the average person to prove their capability.[33] Many adolescents with disabilities have not had part-time jobs. Gleuckauf and Quittner[34] cite many barriers facing young people and, according to Strax,[14] many people are turned away from jobs just because they have a disability. According to his findings fewer than 20% of people with disabilities who are of employment age are in fact employed.

The adolescents did not articulate these same concerns about the future, but they did indicate that they wanted jobs and felt that it was important to get a job. In a study by Polger, King, MacKinnon, Cathers and Havens,[35] having a job and living on one's own were two of the key elements identified as being important to adolescents.

Issues of vulnerability were mentioned often and reflect parents' level of anxiety about their adolescents in the community. Westcott[36] in 1991, and the Institute for the Prevention of Child Abuse in 1995[37] reported that children with disabilities are at an increased risk for abuse. This is also supported by the findings at the Children's Issues Guidance Forum.[33] They found that sexual abuse of women and girls with disabilities occurred more frequently than with other females. The reasons for this increased vulnerability are many-faceted and have been discussed by several authors.[31,34,38-41] Winter and DeSimone[24] believe that the parental urge to protect children from harm is greater when the children have a disability, but the fact is that these children *are* at greater risk for harm and are more vulnerable. The parental fears articulated through these interviews are well founded.

Some of the issues raised were unique to those with physical disabilities, but many of the concerns identified by both parents and adolescents were not dissimilar to concerns raised by parents and adolescents everywhere. The adolescents were most concerned about the here and now, and parents were more concerned about the implications of the current situation and the underlying factors. This is in keeping with normal family functioning.

The generalizability of the results of this study is limited by the small sample size. Further research continuing to explore the perceived needs of adolescents and their parents is recommended.

Many needs have been identified in the provision of rehabilitation services to adolescents. Programmatic changes may be necessary to ensure that these needs are met. The uniqueness of adolescents with disabilities needs to be addressed and the partnership of the adolescents in the rehabilitation process must be acknowledged and allowed to flourish.

REFERENCES

1. Professional Advisory Committee of the Association of Treatment Centres of Ontario & The Neurodevelopmental Clinical Research Unit. *A Perspective on Family-centred Service*. Hamilton, Ont.; 1995.

2. Bailey DB, McWilliam PJ, Winton PJ. Building family-centered practices in early intervention: a team-based model for change. *Infants Young Child*. 1992; 5(1):73-82.

3. Kolobe THA. Working with families of children with disabilities. *Pediatr Phys Ther*. 1992; 4:57-63.

4. Leviton A, Mueller M, Kauffman C. The family-centered consultation model: practical applications for professionals. *Infants Young Child*. 1992; 4(3):1-8.

5. Shelton TL, Stepanek JS. *Family-centered Care for Children Needing Specialized Health and Developmental Services*, 3rd ed. Bethesda, MD: Association for the Care of Children's Health; 1994.

6. Barrett-Lennard GT. The client-centered system: a developmental perspective. In: Turner FJ, ed. *Social Work Treatment: Interlocking Theoretical Approaches*. New York, NY: The Free Press, A Division of Macmillan Publishing Co. Inc.; 1974:181-328.

7. Allen DA, Hudd SS. Are we professionalizing parents? Weighing the benefits and pitfalls. *Mental Retardation*. 1987; 25(3):133-139.

8. Bazyk S. Changes in attitudes and beliefs regarding parent participation and home programs: an update. *Am J Occup Ther.* 1989; 43:723-728.

9. Cadman D, Goldsmith C, Bashim P. Values, preferences, and decisions in the care of children with developmental disabilities. *Dev Behav Pediatr.* 1984; 5(2):60-64.

10. Dunst CJ, Trivette CM, Boyd K, Brookfield J. Help-giving practices and the self-efficacy appraisals of parents. In: Dunst CJ, Trivette CM, Deal YAG, eds. *Supporting and Strengthening Families (Vol.1): Methods, Strategies and Practices.* Cambridge, MA: Brookline Books; 1994:212-220.

11. Hostler SL. Family-centered care. *Pediatr Clin North Am.* 1989; 38;1545-1560.

12. Group for the Advancement of Psychiatry. *Normal Adolescence: Its Dynamics and Impact.* New York, NY: Formulated by the Committee on Adolescence. Vol VI, Report No. 68, Feb. 1968.

13. Hostler SL, Gressard RP, Hassler CR, Linden PG. Adolescent autonomy project: transition skills for adolescents with physical disability. *Child Health Care.* 1989; 18(1):12-18.

14. Strax TE. Psychological issues faced by adolescents and young adults with disabilities. *Pediatr Ann.* 1991; 20(9):507-511.

15. Mulcahey MJ. Returning to school after a spinal cord injury: perspectives from four adolescents. *Am J Occup Ther.* 1992; 46: 305-312.

16. Law M, Baptiste S, Carswell A, McColl MA, Polatajko H, Pollock N. *Canadian Occupational Performance Measure.* 2nd ed. Toronto, Ont: The Canadian Association of Occupational Therapists; 1994.

17. The Canadian Association of Occupational Therapists and The Health Services Directorate, Health Services and Promotion Branch, Health & Welfare, Canada. *Occupational Therapy Guidelines for Client-centred Practice.* Toronto, Ont: The Canadian Association of Occupational Therapists in co-operation with Health & Welfare Canada and the Canadian Government Publishing Centre, Supply and Services, Canada; 1991.

18. Blum RW, Resnick MD, Nelson R, St. Germaine A. Family and peer issues among adolescents with spina bifida and cerebral palsy. *Pediatrics.* 1991; 88: 280-285.

19. King GA, Shultz IZ, Steel K, Gilpin M, Cathers T. Self-evaluation and self-concept of adolescents with physical disabilities. *Am J Occup Ther.* 1993; 47: 132-140.

20. Pollock N, Stewart D. A survey of activity patterns and vocational readiness of young adults with physical disabilities. *Can J Rehabil.* 1990; 4(1):17-26.

21. Richardson SA, Hastorf AH, Dornbush SM. Effects of physical disability on a child's description of himself. *Child Dev.* 1964; 35:893-907.

22. Sinnema G. Resilience among children with special health-care needs and among their families. *Pediatr Ann.* 1991; 20(9):483-486.

23. Stanwyck DJ. Self-esteem through the life span. *Family and Community Health.* 1983; 6(2):11-28.

24. Winter M, DeSimone D. I'm a person, not a wheelchair! Problems of disabled adolescents. In: RL Jones, ed. *Reflections on Growing Up Disabled.* Reston, VA: The Council for Exceptional Children; 1983.

25. Hansen J. *Social self-concept in children with cerebral palsy: its dynamics and impact.* Unpublished manuscript. Toronto: Hugh MacMillan Rehabilitation Centre; 1995.

26. Minde KK. Coping styles of 34 adolescents with cerebral palsy. *Am J Psychiatry.* 1978; 135:1344-1349.

27. Skrtic TM, Summers JA, Brotherson MJ, Turnbull AP. Severely handicapped children and their brothers and sisters. In: Blacher J, ed. *Severely Handicapped Young Children and their Families. Research in Review.* Orlando, FL: Academic Press, Inc.; 1984:215-246.

28. Wallander JL, Varni JW, Babani L, Banis HT, Wilcox KT. Children with chronic physical disorders: maternal reports of their psychological adjustment. *J Pediatr Psychol.* 1988; 13:187-212.

29. Wallander JL, Feldman WS, Varni JW. Physical status and psychosocial adjustment in children with spina bifida. *J Pediatr Psychol.* 1989; 14:89-102.

30. Kokkonen J, Saukkonen AL, Timonen E, Serlo W, Kinnunen P. Social outcome of handicapped children as adults. *Dev Med Child Neurol.* 1991; 33:1095-1100.

31. Schor DP. Sex and sexual abuse in developmentally disabled adolescents. *Sem Adolescent Med.* 1987; 3(1):1-7.

32. Thomas D. *The Social Psychology of Childhood Disability.* London, UK: Methuen & Co. Ltd.; 1978.

33. Ontario Advisory Council on Disability Issues. *Children's Issues Guidance Forum Vol. IV.* Toronto: Publications, Ontario, Ont; 1995.

34. Glueckauf RL, Quittner AL. Facing physical disability as a young adult: psychological issues and approaches. In: Eisenberg MG, Sutkin LC, Jansen MA, eds. *Chronic Illness and Disability Through the Life Span. Effects on Self and Family.* New York, NY: Springer Publishing Company; 1984:176-183.

35. Polgar JM, King G, MacKinnon E, Cathers T, Havens L. *How adolescents with disabilities view success in life.* Presented at the annual conference of The Association of Treatment Centres of Ontario; 1995; Toronto, Ont, Canada.

36. Westcott H. The abuse of disabled children: a review of the literature. *Child Care, Health Dev.* 1991; 17:243-258.

37. The Institute for the Prevention of Child Abuse. Vulnerable children. *Connection.* 1995; 4. Toronto, Ontario.

38. Gaze H. Unspeakable acts. *Nursing Times.* 1992; 88(8):14-15.

39. Laurent C. Trust betrayed. *Nursing Times.* 1993; 89(10):20.

40. Trevelyan J. When it's difficult. *Nursing Times.* 1988; 32:16-17.

41. National Center for Youth with Disabilities. Adolescents with chronic illness and disability: reconsidering a generation of youth, research and knowledge. *Connections. The Newsletter of the National Center for Youth with Disabilities.* 1994; 4(4).

Family-Centred Functional Therapy
for Children with Cerebral Palsy:
An Emerging Practice Model

Mary Law
Johanna Darrah
Nancy Pollock
Gillian King
Peter Rosenbaum
Dianne Russell
Robert Palisano
Susan Harris
Robert Armstrong
Joe Watt

Mary Law, PhD, OT(C), is Director, NCRU, Associate Professor, School of Rehabilitation Science, McMaster University, Hamilton, ON, and an occupational therapist. Johanna Darrah, PhD, PT, is Assistant Professor, University of Alberta at Edmonton, AL. Nancy Pollock, MSc, OT(C), is Assistant Clinical Professor, McMaster University, Hamilton. Gillian King, PhD, is NCRU Investigator, McMaster University, Hamilton and Research Director, Thames Valley Children's Centre, London, ON. Peter Rosenbaum, MD, FRCP(C), is Developmental Pediatrician, NCRU Investigator, and Professor, Department of Pediatrics, McMaster University, Hamilton. Dianne Russell, MSc, is Research Coordinator, NCRU, McMaster University, Hamilton. Robert Palisano, PhD, PT, is Associate Professor, Hahnemann-Allegheny University, Philadelphia, PA, USA. Susan Harris, PhD, PT, is Associate Professor, University of British Columbia at Vancouver, BC. Robert Armstrong, MD, is Associate Professor, University of British Columbia at Vancouver. Joe Watt, MD, is Associate Professor, University of Alberta at Edmonton.

Address correspondence to: Mary Law, Neurodevelopmental Clinical Research Unit, McMaster University, Building T-16, 1280 Main Street West, Hamilton, ON, Canada L8S 4K1.

[Haworth co-indexing entry note]: "Family-Centred Functional Therapy for Children with Cerebral Palsy: An Emerging Practice Model." Law, Mary et al. Co-published simultaneously in *Physical & Occupational Therapy in Pediatrics* (The Haworth Press, Inc.) Vol. 18, No. 1, 1998, pp. 83-102; and: *Family-Centred Assessment and Intervention in Pediatric Rehabilitation* (ed: Mary Law) The Haworth Press, Inc., 1998, pp. 83-102. Single or multiple copies of this article are available for a fee from The Haworth Document Delivery Service [1-800-342-9678, 9:00 a.m. - 5:00 p.m. (EST). E-mail address: getinfo@haworthpressinc.com].

SUMMARY. In this paper we describe the development and initial evaluation of a family-centred functional approach to therapy for young children with cerebral palsy. The family-centred functional therapy approach is based on theoretical concepts from family-centred service and a systems approach to motor development. Principles of this approach include an emphasis on functional performance, and providing therapy when movement behaviors are amenable to change. Therapy focuses on identifying and changing performance constraints in the task, the child or the environment. Four initial studies were completed to develop and evaluate the feasibility of the family-centred functional therapy approach. Results indicate that children receiving this approach improve in functional performance over the course of intervention. Development of the therapy approach needs to continue to enable therapists to develop methods to identify a broader range of factors that enable or constrain task performance. Further development of specific therapeutic strategies is also required, particularly strategies that focus on changing the task or the environment around the child as a means to improve performance. *[Article copies available for a fee from The Haworth Document Delivery Service: 1-800-342-9678. E-mail address: getinfo@haworthpressinc.com]*

Cerebral palsy in children is associated with *impairments* (e.g., in muscle tone, strength, reflexes, range of motion) which are often accompanied by significant *disabilities* (e.g., in dressing, feeding, functional mobility) which, in turn, may lead to *handicap* (e.g., in playing, participating in school).[1] Children with cerebral palsy receive physical therapy and occupational therapy to facilitate motor development and to enhance independence in movement, self-care, play and leisure.

The most common therapy currently used is based on a 'neurodevelopmental' approach.[2-4] In this approach, intervention focuses on improving motor-based activities by changing the child's underlying impairments in motor control through the inhibition and integration of primitive postural patterns and the facilitation of more normal quality of movement.[2] During the past decade, the empirical efficacy of this approach to improve the abilities as well as impairments of young children with cerebral palsy has been widely questioned.[5-9]

Concepts emerging from a systems approach to motor development, and a family-centred approach to services, have led people to consider alternate ways of conceptualizing motor development and intervention to enhance the functional abilities of children with cerebral palsy.[10-14] In such an approach, the focus of intervention is on improving motor-based activities which a child is ready to accomplish through changing identified constraints in the child, task or environment. The purpose of this paper is to describe the development and initial evaluation of such a family-centred functional approach to therapy for young children with cerebral palsy.

LITERATURE REVIEW

Neurodevelopmental Therapy

The neurodevelopmental treatment approach (NDT) remains the predominant method of therapy for young children with cerebral palsy.[3] Occupational therapists and physical therapists are, however, beginning to question this approach, suggesting that the carryover of facilitated normal movement patterns into functional activities is limited.[13,14] Horn and associates,[15] however, tested a combined NDT and behavioral approach with four children with cerebral palsy and found that identified movement components of specific actions (e.g., neck flexion in supine to side rolling) were achieved and did generalize to other settings. In contrast to these findings, a recent crossover trial comparing increased NDT (relative to previous frequency of therapy) to occupational therapy focussed on functional goals, found no evidence of carryover of the treatment effect of NDT on hand function activities either immediately following therapy or 3 months later.[16]

Recent research challenges a hierarchical approach to motor development. For example, Horowitz and Sharby[17] and Fetters et al.[18] have demonstrated that proximal and distal movement control can develop at the same time. We could find no substantive evidence that inhibition of primitive reflex patterns promotes motor development. In fact, research suggests that the disappearance of the stepping reflex in normal development is not the result of maturation of the higher-level nervous system mechanisms but rather is due to the musculoskeletal limitations imposed by the increase in weight of infants between birth and 2 months of age.[19,20] One of the aims of an NDT approach is to decrease muscle tone through inhibition of primitive reflexes. Recent research, however, has indicated that increased tone, as well as postural difficulties, originates as much as or more from biochemical and biomechanical changes than from neural activity.[21] The results of selective dorsal rhizotomy surgery suggest that spasticity alone is an insufficient explanation for abnormal movement patterns.[22] For example, a current focus of research is whether strengthening should be a primary focus of therapy.[23,24]

Clinical evaluation studies have also raised questions about the efficacy of this therapy approach. Nine group comparison studies of NDT-based therapy for children with cerebral palsy have been conducted over the past 20 years. In these studies, the NDT approach has been compared to no therapy,[25] functional therapy,[16,26-28] infant stimulation,[29] Vojta therapy,[30] and differing intensities of therapy.[16,31,32] The results of these trials are mixed with four demonstrating no difference between approaches,[16,26,29,32] three supporting an NDT approach,[27,28,33] and two supporting alternate interventions.[30,31] Studies employing randomized clinical trials have generally produced results that do not support the efficacy of the NDT approach in reducing disability and handicap.[33]

Many of these studies have been criticized because they have not measured what are believed to be the effects of an NDT approach on impairments as well as on disability and handicap. The results of single-case studies have indicated that an NDT approach does have a short-term effect on impairments such as grasp and release patterns,[34,35] movement smoothness and speed,[36] and postural patterns and quality of movement.[3] Whether changes in impairment lead automatically to changes in functional performance is uncertain.[37]

Family-Centred Service

Family-centred service, a philosophy of service provision, is a term which arose from early intervention programs in the United States. In family-centred service, a particular emphasis is on the right of each family to make autonomous decisions. The relationship between the family and professionals is a partnership in which the families define the priorities for therapeutic intervention and, with the therapist, help to direct the intervention process.[12] In working with families, therapists emphasize parent education to enable parents to make informed choices about the therapeutic needs of their child.[38] Therapeutic intervention is based on families' visions and values. Families' roles, interests, the environments in which they live and their culture are recognized as important in a therapy process.[39] Emphasis is placed on the individualization of both the assessment and the intervention process. Therapy is seen as a dynamic process in which service providers and parents work together as partners to define the therapeutic needs of the child with a disability. Services are designed to fit the needs of the families, rather than the families fitting the services or intervention philosophies that are already predetermined by professionals.[40]

A Systems Approach to Motor Development

The systems theoretical framework has been used in various disciplines including chemistry, biology, meteorology, sociology and physics.[20] A systems approach to motor development is based on the concept that goal-directed or task-oriented motor behavior emerges through the interaction and self-organization of many subsystems and that a behavior can be greater than the sum of the individual parts.[20] The framework for this theory as applied to motor development was inspired by the work of Bernstein[41] and principles derived from the physics of motion and change.[42] Bernstein rejected the idea that all muscles were specifically controlled by the cerebral cortex, the traditional 'top-down' approach to motor skills. Instead, he postulated that the cortex controlled muscle groups rather than individual muscles and that the activity of groups of muscles, bones and tendons can modulate motor behavior without receiving instructions from the cerebral cortex.

The systems approach to motor development emerges from a functional rather than a structural framework. The CNS is seen as one of many systems that influence the development of motor function. Other systems include the child's environments as well as the task itself.[43] This framework represents an ecological approach in that a child's functional performance is dependent on the interactions among the child's inherent and emerging skills, the environment in which the task is performed, and the characteristics of the desired task.

When applied to motor development, the key assumptions of this approach are: non-linearity of development; the importance of the context in which a task is performed; self-organization; the effect of periods of change; and constraints on performance. Non-linearity implies that a small change in any subsystem, occurring at a critical stage, can effect a large change in motor behavior. This idea is in contrast to the traditional assumption that motor development depends on the maturation of the CNS. For example, Thelen and Fisher[19] have explained the disappearance of primary stepping as caused by a critical change in the fat to muscle ratio in thigh muscles, resulting in lack of strength to continue stepping in an upright position, as opposed to the more traditional explanation, neurointegration of this reflex. Furthermore, Nashner and McCollum[44] demonstrated that postural responses are dependent on the type of external perturbation as well as the task being performed. Motor strategies self-organize to enable performance of tasks in the most efficient manner. This belief contrasts with the assumption that 'normal' patterns of movement are best for children with cerebral palsy and challenges therapists to reconsider the efficiency of 'abnormal' movement patterns such as bunny-hopping, commando crawling or W-sitting. Are these patterns of movement abnormal or innovative, counter-productive or adaptive?

According to systems theory, periods of instability represent times when movement behaviors are particularly amenable to change. These are the best times to intervene to introduce new movement strategies for a child who is having difficulty making change. Specific factors may encourage or hinder the emergence of motor functions in children with cerebral palsy.[45] *Child* constraints are limitations imposed on motor behaviors by the physical, psychosocial and neurologic characteristics of the child. The integrity of the CNS, biomechanical limitations and motivation are examples of this type of constraint. *Environmental* factors which can constrain the ability to perform a motor task include physical, social, and cultural factors. One example of a physical constraint is gravity, while a social constraint could be parents' lack of reinforcement of a motor behavior. *Task* constraints refer to restrictions on motor behavior imposed by the nature of the task. For example, the size and shape of a spoon will influence the form of a child's grasp, and the height of the table will influence the strategy an infant uses to pull to standing. Any factor or combination of factors from any of these three areas can encourage or hinder the emergence of new motor abilities, depending on its interaction with other critical subsystems.

DEVELOPMENT OF A FAMILY-CENTRED FUNCTIONAL APPROACH TO THERAPY

Our research team has used concepts from a systems approach to motor development, along with the emerging emphasis on family-centredness, to develop a family-centred functional intervention approach for children with cerebral palsy. The following clinical principles define this approach:

1. PROMOTE FUNCTIONAL PERFORMANCE: Function (activity and context) should direct behavior. The goal in therapy is to enable a child to accomplish an identified task, rather than to promote change in an impairment or developmental sequence, or change the way in which a task is accomplished to make it more 'normal.'
2. IDENTIFY PERIODS OF CHANGE: The optimal time to intervene is when a child is trying to do a new task or to do a task in a different way. The child must be motivated to accomplish a task. A young child's parents are the best people to identify when a child is trying to perform the task.
3. IDENTIFY AND CHANGE THE PRIMARY CONSTRAINTS IN THE TASK, CHILD AND/OR ENVIRONMENT THAT PREVENT ACHIEVEMENT OF THE TASK: Parts of tasks or the environment can be changed (e.g., different toy sizes; less noise). Change in a child's abilities (e.g., strength) can

also be targeted during intervention. Tasks incorporated into the daily routine of the child provide increased opportunity to find solutions for functional motor challenges.

4. ENCOURAGE PRACTICE: Young children must practice a newly found motor skill. Practice of activities is the rule for children without disabilities developing any new skill. Tasks should be practiced in a variety of environments which facilitate completion of the task and promote the flexible use of movement strategies.

INITIAL STUDIES OF THE FAMILY-CENTRED FUNCTIONAL APPROACH

Four studies have been completed to develop and evaluate the feasibility of a family-centred functional therapy approach. These studies have focussed on (1) the determination of current practice patterns, (2) family-centred methods to identify functional goals, (3) methods to identify constraints for performance, and (4) an initial evaluation of the family-centred functional approach with 12 children. The first three studies will be described briefly, with the remainder of the paper addressing the pilot results of use of the family-centred functional approach.

I. Current Practice Patterns

To determine patterns of current intervention for children with cerebral palsy, a survey was sent to 82 therapists working in children's rehabilitation centres in three Canadian provinces. The response rate was 100%. Survey respondents were presented with a clinical scenario and asked to describe their goals and intervention approaches. Physical therapists primarily cited mobility (78%) and ambulation (38%) goals and occupational therapists most frequently cited self-care (76%), fine motor skills (62%) and play skills (45%). When asked about predominant intervention approaches or techniques, the NDT approach and techniques were cited by 64% of the physical therapists and 72% of the occupational therapists. The results of this survey indicate that the majority of these therapists use NDT principles as the primary basis for their intervention approach with young children with cerebral palsy. These findings are similar to another recent practice survey.[3]

II. Family-Centred Methods to Identify Therapy Goals

In the second study with two children, ages 3.5 and 4 years, we tested the feasibility of using the Canadian Occupational Performance Measure

(COPM) to enable parents to identify tasks that their children were trying to accomplish.[46] The COPM is an individualized client and family-centred measure administered in an interview format. Parents are asked to identify tasks that their children are trying to perform and to provide ratings (using a 1-10 scale) of the importance of each task. We also used this study to test and further develop an approach to identifying performance constraints. The findings indicated that, through the COPM interview, the parents were easily able to identify tasks their children were trying to accomplish. Therapists and parents were also able to identify many of the performance constraints that influenced task performance. From these experiences, a more formal protocol for identifying constraints was developed.

III. Identifying Readiness and Performance Constraints

A third study was designed to evaluate the ability of the parent/therapist team to identify accurately constraints preventing the child's success at a new motor behavior. The task of walking independently was selected; a child was considered ready to walk if he or she was beginning to stand alone. Four children (ages 2-2.9 years) were identified as being in this period of change. Findings indicated that pre-defining criteria to identify readiness for a task are not beneficial. Instead, parent-identified goals, confirmed by therapist's observations, were more realistic and relevant. For example, instead of using a restricted criterion such as emerging dorsiflexion balance reactions for identifying readiness for standing alone and walking, parents' descriptions of the child 'letting go more' and 'cruising more than crawling,' when verified by therapist observation, were more valid than constrained criteria at the level of impairment. More than one limitation preventing performance was usually present. Often, these constraints were not likely to be changed by 'hands-on' intervention by the therapist. For example, intervention to encourage independent standing and walking was initiated with one child clearly in transition for these skills. Intervention consisted of regular periods of encouraging walking in a playground near home by methods other than holding his hands (using a broomstick, a big ball, holding at his pelvis). Outcome was measured by the percentage of time during 30 minutes of observation when he was cruising instead of crawling. During intervention, cruising time increased from the three baseline observations; however, two weeks after intervention ceased, cruising percentage had reverted back to pre-intervention levels. He subsequently walked independently 4 weeks later, when he was ready to do it. In these instances, intervention to change only one factor (e.g., lack of balance) may not be effective and therapists may be most effective by providing developmental education to the parents so that they can encourage their children in trying new motor tasks. Motivation of the child was confirmed to be a significant prerequisite for success in achieving the new motor task.

IV. Pilot Study of the Family-Centred Functional Approach

The purpose of this study was to complete a pilot evaluation of the family-centred functional therapy approach with 12 children with cerebral palsy. Questions to be answered during this study included:

1. Could parents identify tasks that their children were trying to accomplish?
2. Are therapists able to identify a broad spectrum of constraints to task performance and the specific treatment strategies that could be used to change identified constraints?
3. Do children receiving this therapy approach improve their functional task performance?

Participants

Twelve participants were selected from children receiving physical therapy and occupational therapy services at three children's rehabilitation centres in Alberta and Ontario, Canada (see Table 1 for demographic information). The *inclusion* criteria were: diagnosis of cerebral palsy (hemi-

TABLE 1. Description of Study Participants

Age:	One year	2
	-Two years	6
	Three years	3
	Four years	1
Sex:	Male	5
	Female	7
Primary Language:	English	11
	Filipino	1
Preschool Attendance:	Yes	8
	No	4
Primary Caregiver:	Mother	12
Participation in other community programs	Yes	2
	No	10

plegia, quadriplegia or diplegia), based on published diagnostic crite-ria;[47] ability to attend therapy sessions during the study period; and ages 18 months to 5 years. Children having recent or planned surgery (e.g., selective dorsal rhizotomy) that affects motor function were excluded. Parents or guardians of children signed an informed consent prior to study entry.

Study Intervention

An occupational therapist and a physical therapist worked together with each child and family. Motor-based tasks which a child was beginning to do, trying to do differently, or showing an interest in doing but having difficulty accomplishing, were identified by parents using the COPM assessment. Parents and therapists then observed these tasks to confirm that the child was in a period of change. Prerequisites for recommending intervention were that the child had to be identified as trying to do a new task or doing a task in a different way and that the child must be motivated to accomplish the task.

Working with the parents, therapists then identified the constraints in the child, task or environment that were hindering performance of the task, as well as factors that facilitated performance. Constraints were identified through the use of further standardized assessments of the child, observation of task performance and further discussion with parents. Intervention was only provided when the child was interested in trying a task and when constraints were identified for which intervention could be provided.

Intervention focussed on changing the constraints that were judged as most amenable to change. Intervention included opportunities for practice of tasks in context. The expected outcome was functional and environmentally-appropriate movement, without any particular concern for the quality of the movement. For example, if poor balance was identified as preventing a child from sitting and playing, then the aim of intervention could be to help the child achieve that support by a seating modification. If the child chose to sit in a more stable position such as a 'W' sit, that would not be actively discouraged. If a young child was having difficulty in pulling socks on and off, the task was changed by using looser socks. If the difficulty with pulling off socks was due to problems with sitting balance, the environment was changed to provide support for sitting so that the activity could be accomplished. Intervention focussed on changing constraints only for a short time period, after which reassessment occurred. The effects of intervention were always evaluated within the context of achievement of a functional task. Children were encouraged to use any compensatory strategies to achieve functional tasks; therefore, spontaneously chosen movement patterns such as scooting, commando crawling or pulling to standing using arms were encouraged if they were effective, least intrusive, and acceptable to the child.

Parent education and consultation about home programs were provided. This recognizes the importance of practice and repetition in a meaningful context for learning to occur. The focus was on working with parents to identify tasks which the child was trying to do and helping parents to implement changes to factors which were hindering their child from accomplishing a task. Therapy sessions usually took place at the children's rehabilitation centre. Therapists completed a therapy log to indicate the task identified, the constraints to performance, the intervention strategies and attendance at therapy sessions. Table 2 describes examples of the therapy process.

Measurement of Outcome

The outcome measures used in the pilot study included the Gross Motor Function Measure (GMFM),[48] Peabody Developmental Fine Motor Scale (PDMS-FM),[49] Pediatric Evaluation of Disability Inventory (PEDI),[50] and Canadian Occupational Performance Measure (COPM).[47] For the GMFM, only the dimensions that were goal areas for each child (e.g., sitting) were tested. To decrease assessment burden, a randomized schedule was used to ensure that each assessment, other than the COPM, was administered to 6 participants. One GMFM could be collected after intervention. Assessments were performed at baseline and 3 months later and were completed by independent evaluators.

RESULTS

Using the COPM, parents identified from 2 to 8 tasks that they felt that their children were trying to accomplish (total number of tasks = 73). Self-care, mobility and play tasks were identified most frequently (Table 3). Using the importance rating procedure for the COPM, the 5 tasks judged most important by the parents became the targets for intervention (total number of tasks = 59). Children received an average of 10-12 therapy sessions during a 3-month period. Intervention focussed on 2 to 3 tasks at a time. Length of intervention for each task was usually 4 to 6 sessions, but this time frame ranged from 2 to 12 sessions. Child motivation and interest, family support, and the frequency that the task was done were the most frequent factors enabling performance while the child's postural tone, the

TABLE 2. Examples of the Family-Centred Functional Approach

I. Identified Task: To keep up with his older sister by moving his walker more quickly

Area of Analysis	Factors helping task performance	Factors hindering task performance
CHILD	motivation to be with sister cognitive ability	increased tone movement patterns absence of postural reaction
TASK		speed at which task needs to be performed
ENVIRONMENT	encouragement provided by sister layout of his home	walker setup

Intervention Focus:

Adjust angle of seat on walker to position him forward and facilitate movement (not successful)

Investigate power mobility options (parents were interested in focussing on this option and it was successful)

II. Identified Task: To drink from a regular cup and scoop with a spoon

Area of Analysis	Factors helping task performance	Factors hindering task performance
CHILD	postural control in sitting functional use of left arm	attention/endurance associates mother with feeding her
TASK	use of finger foods use of food that she likes use of familiar utensils	new seating
ENVIRONMENT	family eating at same time	younger brother distracting table cluttered

Intervention Focus:

Use familiar toy chair/table; booster chair with back support; mother out of room (not successful)

Use box seat; small cup; towel on table for spills; family eating at same time (successful)

physical demands of the tasks, and gravity and distractions were the most frequent constraints identified in the child, the task, and the environment, respectively (Table 4). Overall, the most frequently identified constraints were in the child; these included tone, balance, strength, interest, and range of motion.

TABLE 3. Summary of Tasks Identified by Parents on the COPM

Task	Number of times identified (N = 79)	Number of times a priority for intervention (N = 43)
Washing/bathing/toiletting	10	4
Walking	9	9
Dressing	9	3
Playing independently	7	4
Sitting	6	6
Feeding	5	2
Communication	5	1
Moving on/off furniture/climbing	5	5
Standing to do activity	4	4
Swimming/other recreation	4	1
Moving on floor (crawling)	3	1
Making numbers/letters	3	1
Cutting with scissors	2	1
Riding a tricycle	1	1

An analysis of the intervention strategies indicated that intervention was provided for 43 of the 59 tasks that were rated as a priority on the COPM. The primary reasons for not providing intervention were lack of time during the 3-month period to address the issue or the timing of intervention was not suitable for the family. In a few cases, the child accomplished the task before intervention was started or further analysis indicated that the child was not yet ready to accomplish the task. In situations where the child was not ready, developmental education was provided to parents. This education focussed on general ideas to promote motor task experiences for their children. Analysis of the intervention provided indicated that the therapeutic focus was primarily on changing factors within the child (N = 31) compared to changing the task (N = 14) or the environment (N = 21).

Results from the outcome evaluation after the intervention indicated that the mean scores for each measure improved over the 3-month study period. Information from the measurement manuals[44,46,47] was used to determine that clinically important change had occurred in the COPM scores, the GMFM, and the PEDI mobility mean scores (Table 5). For these same outcome measures, 11 of the 12 children in the study demonstrated changes that were clinically important. Analysis of the statistical significance of the change scores was not completed because the sample size was small and the purpose of the study was to examine feasibility issues, not intervention effectiveness.

TABLE 4. Summary of Task Constraints and Enabling Factors

	Enabling Factor	# times identified	Constraint	# times identified
CHILD	motivation/interest	43	tone	24
	cognitive ability	10	balance	14
	enjoys tasks	7	strength	12
	motor ability	5	interest	12
	determination	4	range of motion	11
	range of motion	3	abnormal movements	5
	independence	2	motor control	5
	weight of child	1	coordination	4
			primitive reflexes	4
			resistant to change	2
TASK	frequency	14	physical demands	17
	developmental level	6	physical properties of	9
	task demands	6	assistive device	
	equipment available	3	height of furniture	6
	can be done anywhere	3	unfamiliarity	4
	familiarity	2	cognitive demands	3
	water buoyancy	1	do only occasionally	2
	task easy to do in steps	1	position of child required	2
	size of objects	1	energy required	2
	location	1	time required	2
ENVIRONMENT	parent/family support	31	gravity	8
	assistive devices	8	distractions	7
	role models	7	limited space	5
	furniture	5	family expectations	5
	parents think it is	4	uneven surface	4
	important		physical demand on	3
	quiet	3	family	
	suitable space	3	furniture position	3
	toy availability	2	assistance not available	3
	parent absent	1	nature of assistive device	3
	stimulating	1	task location	3
	community program	1	weather	1
			cold water	1
			parent absent	1

DISCUSSION

The family-centred functional approach to therapy, as evaluated in this pilot study, appears to have potential to facilitate change in motor performance in young children with cerebral palsy. Children receiving intervention in the pilot study made changes in performance that were observable and clinically meaningful over the course of the study period. Because this

TABLE 5. Mean Change Between Pre- and Post-Evaluation on Outcome Measures

	Baseline Evaluation Mean (Standard deviation)	After Intervention Mean (Standard deviation)	Mean Change
COPM (n = 12) (Score ranges from 1-10)			
Performance	3.31 (1.13)	6.25 (1.16)	2.94
Satisfaction	3.40 (1.70)	6.60 (2.00)	3.20
GMFM (n = 5) (% of 100)	12.9 (10.40)	30.58 (16.88)	17.68
PEDI (n = 6) (Raw score sums for each domain)			
Self-care	20.67 (10.75)	23.67 (13.60)	3.00
Mobility	14.50 (6.72)	20.33 (9.95)	5.83
Social	23.17 (12.24)	26.00 (9.63)	2.83
PDMS-FM (n = 6) (total raw score)	141.33 (18.68)	151.67 (18.76)	10.34

study had no control group, separating the effects of intervention from the effects of maturation is not possible; but the changes documented support the value of continuing to develop and evaluate this therapy approach.

Therapy assessment and intervention in the family-centred functional approach begins with and focuses on parent-identified goals for their children. Parents in this study were able to identify tasks in which their children were showing interest or were trying to perform. In fact, results from our studies indicated that parents identify these tasks more easily than therapists. Because several times tasks were identified but found subsequently not to be ready for change, further work defining the concept of task readiness, and how to enable both parents and therapists to identify readiness, is required. Feedback from the therapists indicated that they found that the procedure of identifying goals, as well as enabling and constraining performance factors, was a useful structure for the therapy process. These initial procedures of the intervention appeared to be learned and applied by the therapists in this study; however, the number of enabling or constraining factors identified could be broadened to include a wider range of factors. For example, many aspects of cognition, such as memory, problem-solving, imitation and learning style can influence performance. Similarly, environmental factors can also include temporal, economic, cultural and educational factors. A more comprehensive understanding of these many factors that can influence childhood task performance needs to be developed.

Therapists reported that they encountered the most difficulty with the next step of the therapy process, that of choosing the initial intervention focus. They had difficulty working with the parents to select the most appropriate factor(s) to address in order to facilitate change in performance. Several reasons may account for this difficulty. First, some of the identified factors are clearly challenging or impossible to change (e.g., gravity, muscle tone). Second, for those factors that may be changeable (e.g., attention, parent/child interaction), specific strategies for change are not always clear. Further work is required to develop these strategies. A third reason may be a difficulty in changing one's practice style. The focus of the intervention strategies in this study supports this reasoning. We had expected the intervention to focus more on changing task or environmental factors because these factors are often easier to change than those present in the child. The results of the therapy analysis, however, indicated that the focus was primarily on changing factors within the child. Prior to the pilot study, a one-day workshop on the therapy approach was held for all participating therapists. This, along with the paucity of specific therapy strategies, may not be enough to facilitate practice change. Further research will focus on the development of therapeutic strategies and training methods for implementation of this approach.

The development of any new or modified approach to intervention is challenging. In this situation, it is particularly difficult because some of the assessment of task performance and interventions used may be very similar to what many therapists do already. The question then becomes—is this approach different, or is it describing therapy that is already in use? The answer to that question is complex. Our initial survey of therapy practice indicated that an NDT approach is still predominant in intervention for children with cerebral palsy; however, what therapists considered to be an NDT approach is not clear from our survey. Is it an approach to therapy based on a hierarchical, neuromaturational model which emphasizes the facilitation of normal patterns of movement, or is it a combination of this and other added techniques that are collectively called an NDT approach?

Although similarities to an NDT approach exist in the specific intervention strategies used in the family-centred functional approach, particularly when the focus is on changing child-related factors, many differences are also apparent. The underlying theoretical assumptions of the family-centred functional approach are based on a systems approach to motor development that is non-hierarchical. Family-defined functional tasks are the focus of intervention. The primary goal of therapy is task accomplishment, with no particular emphasis on movement quality. Finally, the focus of intervention is broader, with a greater emphasis on changing task and environmental factors which are constraining task performance.

Research is continuing to develop further the family-centred functional approach to intervention. A need exists to generate a more extensive list of factors that have the potential to influence task performance, to define how these factors can best be identified as enabling or constraining performance, and to determine which factors are most easily modified. Specific therapeutic strategies to modify constraining factors require continued development so that therapists will be able and comfortable to enlarge their repertoire of intervention strategies. Finally, the efficacy of this approach needs continued evaluation to determine whether it is useful as a model for intervention for young children with cerebral palsy.

AUTHOR NOTE

The authors wish to thank the children and their parents who participated in these studies. They also thank the therapists at the Children's Developmental Rehabilitation Program of the Hamilton Health Sciences Corporation, Glenrose Rehabilitation Centre, and Lansdowne Children's Centre for their support and participation.

This research was funded by the United Cerebral Palsy Research and Educational Foundation and is part of the research program of the Neurodevelopmental Clinical Research Unit at McMaster University.

REFERENCES

1. World Health Organization (WHO). *International Classification of Impairment, Disability and Handicap.* Geneva, Switzerland: WHO; 1980.

2. Bly L. A historical and current view of the basis of NDT. *Pediatr Phys Ther.* 1991;3:131-135.

3. DeGangi GA, Royeen CB. Current practice among Neurodevelopmental Treatment Association members. *Am J Occup Ther.* 1994;48:803-809.

4. VanSant AF. Neurodevelopmental Treatment and pediatric physical therapy: a commentary. *Pediatr Phys Ther.* 1991;3:137-141.

5. Embrey DG. Efficacy studies in children with cerebral palsy: focus on upper extremity function. *Phys Occup Ther Pediatr.* 1993;12(4):89-95.

6. Harris SR. Early intervention: does developmental therapy make a difference? *Topics in Early Childhood Special Education.* 1988;7(4):20-32.

7. Palisano RJ. Research on the effectiveness of Neurodevelopmental Treatment. *Pediatr Phys Ther.* 1991;3:143-148.

8. Parette HP, Hendricks MD, Rock SL. Efficacy of therapeutic intervention intensity with infants and young children with cerebral palsy. *Infants Young Child.* 1991;4:1-19.

9. Parette HP, Hourcade J. A review of therapeutic intervention research on gross and fine motor progress in young children with cerebral palsy. *Am J Occup Ther.* 1984;38:462-468.

10. Canadian Association of Occupational Therapists. *Occupational Therapy Guidelines for Client-centred Practice.* Toronto, ON: CAOT Publications; 1991.

11. Damiano DL. Reviewing muscle co-contraction: is it a developmental, pathological, or motor control issue? *Phys Occup Ther Pediatr.* 1993;12(1):3-20.

12. Dunst C, Trivette C, Deal A. *Enabling and Empowering Families–Principles and Guidelines for Practice.* Cambridge, MA: Brookline Books, Inc.; 1988.

13. Horak FB. Motor control models underlying neurologic rehabilitation of posture in children. In: Forssberg H, Hirschfeld H, eds. *Movement Disorders in Children.* New York, NY: Karger; 1992, 21-30.

14. Piper MC, Darrah J. *Motor Assessment of the Developing Infant.* Philadelphia, PA: WB Saunders; 1994.

15. Horn EM, Warren SF, Jones HA. An experimental analysis of a neurobehavioral motor intervention. *Dev Med Child Neurol.* 1995;37:697-714.

16. Law M, Russell D, Pollock N, Rosenbaum P, Walter S, King G. A comparison of intensive neurodevelopmental therapy and casting and regular occupational therapy for young children with cerebral palsy. *Dev Med Child Neurol.* In press.

17. Horowitz L, Sharby N. Development of prone extension postures in healthy infants. *Phys Ther.* 1988;68:32-39.

18. Fetters L, Fernandez B, Cermak S. The relationship of proximal and distal components in the development of reaching. *Phys Ther.* 1988;68:839.

19. Thelen E, Fisher DM. Newborn stepping: an explanation for a "disappearing reflex." *Dev Psychol.* 1982;18:760-775.

20. Thelen E, Kelso JAS, Fogel A. Self-organizing systems and infant motor development. *Dev Rev.* 1987;7:39-65.

21. Tardieu G, Tardieu C, Colbeau-Justin P, Lespargo A. Muscle hypoextensibility in children with cerebral palsy. II: Therapeutic implications. *Arch Phys Med Rehabil.* 1982;63:103-107.

22. Giuliani CA. Dorsal rhizotomy for children with cerebral palsy: support for concepts of motor control. *Phys Ther.* 1991;71:248-259.

23. MacPhail HEA, Kramer JR. Effects of isokinetic strengthening on functional ability and walking efficiency of adolescents with cerebral palsy. *Dev Med Child Neurol.* 1995;37:763-775.

24. Damiano DL, Kelly LE, Vaughn CL. Effects of quadriceps femoris muscle strengthening on crouch gait of children with spastic diplegia. *Phys Ther.* 1995;75:658-667.

25. Wright T, Nicholson J. Physiotherapy for the spastic child: an evaluation. *Dev Med Child Neurol.* 1973;15:146-163.

26. Carlsen PN. Comparison of two occupational therapy approaches for treating the young cerebral-palsied child. *Am J Occup Ther.* 1975;29:267-272.

27. Scherzer AL, Mike V, Ilson J. Physical therapy as a determinant of change in the cerebral palsied infant. *Pediatrics.* 1976;53:47-52.

28. Sommerfeld D, Fraser BA, Hensinger RN, Beresford CV. Evaluation of physical therapy service for severely mentally impaired students with cerebral palsy. *Phys Ther.* 1981;61:338-344.

29. Palmer FB, Shapiro BK, Wachtal RC, et al. The effects of physical therapy on cerebral palsy: a controlled trial in infants with spastic diplegia. *New Eng J Med.* 1988;318:903-908.

30. D'Avignon M. Early physiotherapy ad modum Vojta or Bobath in infants with suspected neuromotor disturbance. *Neuropediatrics.* 1981;12:232-241.

31. Law M, Cadman D, Rosenbaum P, DeMatteo C, Walter S, Russell D. Neurodevelopmental therapy and upper extremity casting: results of a clinical trial. *Dev Med Child Neurol.* 1991;33:334-340.

32. Mayo NE. The effect of physical therapy for children with motor delay and cerebral palsy. *Am J Phys Med Rehabil.* 1991;70:258-267.

33. Piper MC. Efficacy of physical therapy: rate of motor development in children with cerebral palsy. *Pediatr Phys Ther.* 1990;2:126-130.

34. Barnes KJ. Improving prehension skills of children with cerebral palsy. *Occup Ther J Research.* 1986;6:227-240.

35. Barnes KJ. Direct replication: relationship of upper extremity weight bearing to hand skills of boys with cerebral palsy. *Occup Ther J Research.* 1989; 9:235-242.

36. Kluzik J, Fetters L, Coryell J. Quantification of control: a preliminary study of effects of Neurodevelopmental Treatment on reaching in children with spastic cerebral palsy. *Phys Ther.* 1990;70:65-76.

37. Badley EM, Lee J. Impairment, disability and the ICIDH model I: The relationship between impairment and disability. *Int J Rehabil Med.* 1987;8:113-124.

38. Bazyk S. Changes in attitudes and beliefs regarding parent participation and home programs: an update. *Am J Occup Ther.* 1989;43:723-728.

39. Law M. The environment: a focus for occupational therapy. *Can J Occup Ther.* 1991;58:171-179.

40. Law M, Baptiste S, Mills J. Client-centred practice: what does it mean and does it make a difference? *Can J Occup Ther.* 1995;62:250-257.

41. Bernstein N. *Coordination and Regulation of Movements.* New York, NY: Wiley; 1967.

42. Haken H. *Synergetics, an Introduction: Non-equilibrium Phase Transitions and Self-organization in Physics, Chemistry and Biology.* 3rd ed. New York, NY: Springer-Verlag New York Inc.; 1983.

43. Heriza CB. Motor development: traditional and contemporary theories. In: Lister M, ed. *Contemporary Management of Motor Control Problems: Proceedings of the II-step Conference.* Alexandria, VA: Foundation for Physical Therapy; 1991;99-126.

44. Nashner LM, McCollum G. The organization of human postural movements: a formal basis and experimental synthesis. *Behav Brain Sci.* 1985;8:135-172.

45. Newell KM. Constraints on the development of coordination. In: Wade MG, Whiting HTA, eds. *Motor Development in Children: Aspects of Coordination and Control.* Dordrecht: Martinus Nijhoff; 1985:341-360.

46. Law M, Polatajko H, Pollock N, Carswell A, Baptiste S, McColl M. The Canadian Occupational Performance Measure: results of pilot testing. *Can J Occup Ther.* 1994;61:191-197.

47. McDonald ET. *Treating Cerebral Palsy: For Clinicians by Clinicians.* Austin, TX: Pro-Ed; 1987:1-19.

48. Russell D, Rosenbaum P, Cadman D, Gowland C, Hardy S, Jarvis S. The Gross Motor Function Measure: a means to evaluate the effects of physical therapy. *Dev Med Child Neurol.* 1989;31:341-352.

49. Folio R, Fewell R, DuBose RF. *Peabody Developmental Motor Scales.* Toronto, ON: Teaching Resources Co.; 1983.

50. Haley SM, Coster WJ, Ludlow LH, Haltiwanger J, Andrellos P. *Pediatric Evaluation of Disability Inventory (PEDI). Development, Standardization and Administration Manual.* Boston, MA: New England Medical Center Hospitals; 1992.

Index